Interpreting
Chest X-Rays

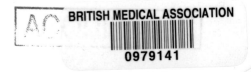

Interpreting Chest X-Rays

Stephen Ellis

Consultant Thoracic Radiologist
St Bartholomew's Hospital and
The London Chest Hospital, London, UK

Scion

© **Scion Publishing Ltd, 2010**

ISBN 978 1 904842 77 4

First published in 2010

A CIP catalogue record for this book is available from the British Library.

Scion Publishing Limited
The Old Hayloft, Vantage Business Park, Bloxham Road, Banbury, Oxfordshire OX16 9UX
www.scionpublishing.com

Important Note from the Publisher

The information contained within this book was obtained by Scion Publishing Limited from sources believed by us to be reliable. However, while every effort has been made to ensure its accuracy, no responsibility for loss or injury whatsoever occasioned to any person acting or refraining from action as a result of information contained herein can be accepted by the authors or publishers.

Although every effort has been made to ensure that all owners of copyright material have been acknowledged in this publication, we would be pleased to acknowledge in subsequent reprints or editions any omissions brought to our attention.

Readers should remember that medicine is a constantly evolving science and while the authors and publishers have ensured that all dosages, applications and practices are based on current indications, there may be specific practices which differ between communities. You should always follow the guidelines laid down by the manufacturers of specific products and the relevant authorities in the country in which you are practising.

Typeset by AM Design, Banbury
Printed by Henry Ling Ltd, Dorchester, UK

Contents

Preface

With the advent of picture archive and communication systems, radiological imaging has become readily accessible to a wide range of healthcare workers who are increasingly taking on extended roles. This book aims to assist not only doctors and medical students, but also the whole range of healthcare workers who are finding the interpretation of the plain chest radiograph (CXR) a routine part of their work.

This is not intended to be an exhaustive text but concentrates on interpretive skills and pattern recognition to enable the reader to understand the pitfalls and clues that will enable them to interpret the CXRs they are likely to encounter in their practice without necessarily having an exhaustive medical knowledge at their fingertips.

S. Ellis

February 2010

Abbreviations

AP	anterior–posterior
A–P	aorto–pulmonary
ARDS	adult respiratory distress syndrome
AXR	abdominal X-ray
CR	computed radiography
CTR	cardio–thoracic ratio
CXR	chest radiograph
DR	digital radiography
HP	hypersensitivity pneumonitis
HRCT	high resolution computed tomography
LAM	lymphangioleiomyomatosis
LCH	Langerhans cell histiocytosis
LLL	left lower lobe
LUL	left upper lobe
NSCLC	non-small cell lung cancer
PA	posterior–anterior
PE	pulmonary embolus
RLL	right lower lobe
RML	right middle lobe
RUL	right upper lobe
SCLC	small cell lung cancer
SOS	satisfaction of search
SPN	solitary pulmonary nodule
SVC	superior vena cava
V/Q	ventilation/perfusion

01 Technique

The challenge in taking a CXR lies in the imaging of structures that vary dramatically in density, from aerated lung to bone. The main techniques are outlined below. The technique chosen will depend on the availability of equipment and the location of the patient; the techniques available in the X-ray department are not readily reproducible on the wards. Ultimately, an X-ray image is the shadow of the structure being X-rayed and therefore a proportion of the X-rays must be 'stopped' by that structure; this occurs by either absorption or scatter. Absorption results in radiation dose and is therefore kept to the minimum necessary to form a diagnostic image; unabsorbed scattered X-rays become a problem if they reach the X-ray film / detector because they result in 'unsharpness', similar to the lack of sharpness of a shadow produced by two lights close together.

1.1 Techniques available

1.1.1 High kV (120–140 kV)

The high kV technique was developed to give a better view of the structures behind the heart and hemi-diaphragms compared to low kV CXR.

Scatter reaching the X-ray film is more of a problem with high kV films and a grid that allows undeviated X-rays through, but absorbs scattered X-rays, is used in the X-ray department to reduce the impact of this; an alternative technique involves moving the X-ray source further from the patient, so the X-rays exposing the film are less divergent, and then introducing an air gap between the patient and the X-ray film so that any scattered X-rays 'miss' the film. Mobile X-rays taken on the ward or in theatre cannot employ grids or air gaps and are done with a low kV.

1.1.2 Low kV (60–80 kV)

The low kV technique produces less scatter and therefore does not require a grid; it is used for mobile X-rays. The disadvantage is that the penetration is poorer than with the high kV technique, resulting in poor visualization of the structures behind the heart and hemi-diaphragms. When a low kV technique was used routinely for departmental X-rays, lateral films were also routinely taken to image these areas of the chest.

1.1.3 Digital CXR

Digital radiography is a fundamentally different way of capturing an X-ray image. The incident X-rays either generate an electrical signal directly on the detector (digital radiography, DR), or generate a latent fluorescence on a plate, which is revealed when exposed to a reading laser beam (computed radiography, CR). The advantage of the latter is that the plates can replace the original film cassettes so that the original X-ray equipment can be used. DR requires dedicated equipment and is therefore more costly to set up, but provides a quicker solution without the need to put plates in a reader after exposure.

The response of the plates to incident X-rays in both techniques is linear (unlike conventional X-ray film), enabling a well-penetrated image to be generated at around 80–85 kV with no requirement for a grid. However, the CXR images produced on a digital system with a high kV (125 kV) and a grid are of particularly good quality and high kV imaging may once again become standard practice for CXRs even on digital systems (*Fig. 1.1*).

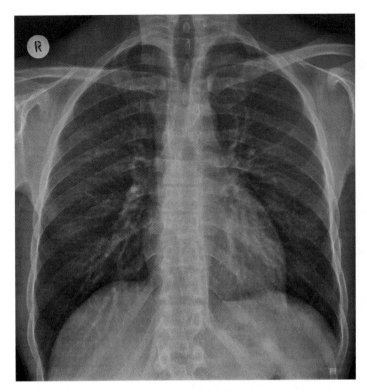

Figure 1.1. Frontal CXR of an adult taken on a digital system using a high kV and a grid.

The clarity of the vessels and the structures behind the heart is extremely good.

1.1.4 PA versus AP

A posterior to anterior (PA) CXR is taken in the radiology department with the patient standing erect in front of and facing the X-ray plate, with the X-ray tube positioned behind the patient.

For patients unable to attend the X-ray department, a mobile technique is used. The X-ray film is placed behind the patient, who is either lying supine or semi-erect holding the plate in position by leaning against it, and the X-ray source is in front, such that the X-rays pass from anterior to posterior (AP).

Due to practical constraints the X-ray source is closer to the X-ray plate for a mobile AP CXR; the X-rays are therefore more divergent (see *Fig. 1.2*) and cause magnification of anterior structures, those furthest from the X-ray plate, such as the heart. Imagine the shadow of a hand cast on a wall by a torch; as the hand is moved further from the wall and closer to the torch, the shadow is magnified.

Although an essential part of the management of the ill patient, mobile AP CXRs should be interpreted with caution.

Figure 1.3 shows the difference in appearance between AP and PA images. Not only does the heart appear enlarged due to the geometry of the AP technique, the conditions under which the AP CXR is taken with the patient sitting result in a less good inspiratory effort. With the patient standing for a PA film the patient is able to put their hands on their hips with their shoulders internally rotated which moves the scapulae such that they do not overlap the lungs on the CXR.

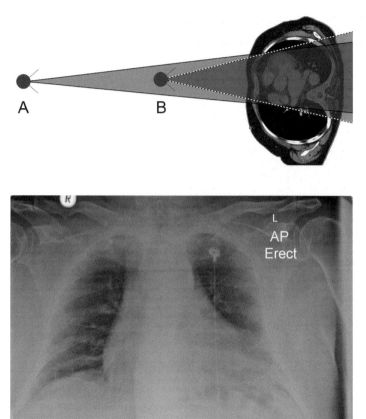

Figure 1.2. Divergent X-rays on a mobile CXR.

A diagrammatic representation of the more divergent X-rays resulting from a shorter distance of the X-ray source (position B) to the patient compared to the longer distance (position A).

(a)

Figures 1.3. Comparison of (a) AP versus (b) PA images.

Compare the AP CXR (a) with the PA CXR (b) performed on the same patient on the same day. Note the alteration in the size of the cardiac silhouette.

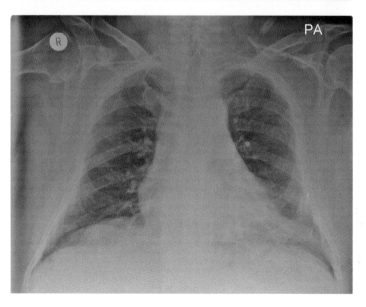

(b)

1.1.5 The lateral CXR

Lateral CXRs are not usually performed because the advent of high kV CXR and subsequently DR has resulted in a PA CXR with good visualization of the previously hidden areas of the chest behind the hemi-diaphragms and the heart.

However, the lateral CXR is not just included here for completeness, because the anterior mediastinum, a blind area on PA CXR, and the contour of the hemi-diaphragms are both better appreciated on lateral CXR (*Fig. 1.4*).

In reality, CT scanning is performed when an abnormality is thought to be present on PA CXR, but the lateral view can be of value in determining:

- whether an abnormality originates from beneath the hemi-diaphragm (i.e. a hernia) obviating the need for a CT scan
- confirming pathology not lying in line with the incident X-rays on a PA film (such as lingula or middle lobe collapse, or loculated fluid in the oblique fissure), which appear on PA CXR as subtle increases in density and can prove difficult to interpret (see *Fig. 1.5*).

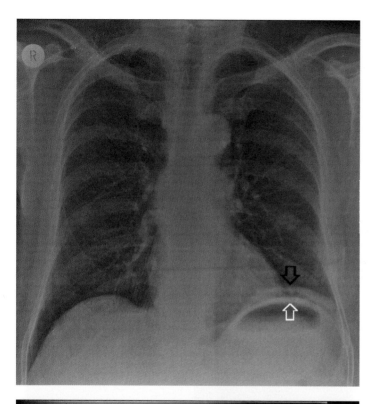

(a)

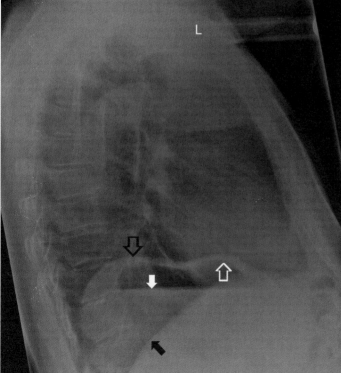

(b)

Figure 1.4. Comparison of (a) PA and (b) lateral CXRs of an adult.

On the frontal CXR (a) there is an odd double contour to the left hemi-diaphragm; the lateral view (b) confirms that this is due to an eventration (open black arrow) of the left hemi-diaphragm (open white arrow), with a fluid/gas-filled fundus of the stomach beneath (white arrow). Note the contour of the right hemi-diaphragm (black arrow).

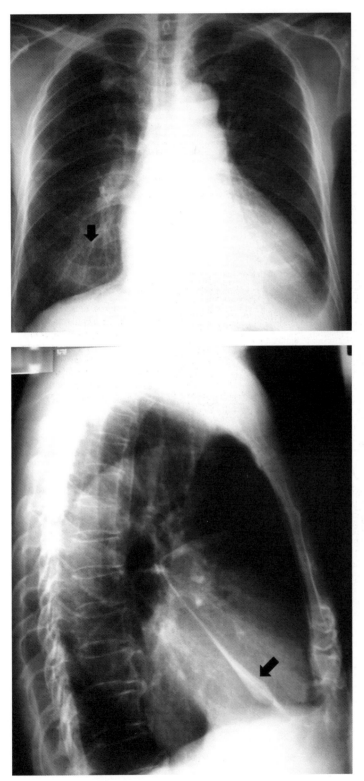

(a)

(b)

Figure 1.5. Frontal (a) and lateral (b) CXRs of an adult with a small left pleural effusion.

On the frontal CXR (a) there is a subtle increase in density in the right lower zone that on the lateral view (b) is shown to be due to loculated fluid in the oblique fissure (black arrow). Note that none of the soft tissue / aerated lung interfaces generated by this fluid are in line with the X-rays of the frontal CXR and therefore do not form a silhouette.

02 Anatomy

A good working knowledge of chest anatomy should enable you, on most occasions, to identify an abnormality and place it in the correct area of the chest. Bear in mind that a CXR is a two-dimensional representation of a three-dimensional structure and, as a result, the CXR includes many overlapping structures.

2.1 Frontal CXR

The main anatomical structures that form the mediastinal silhouette are summarised in *Figure 2.1*.

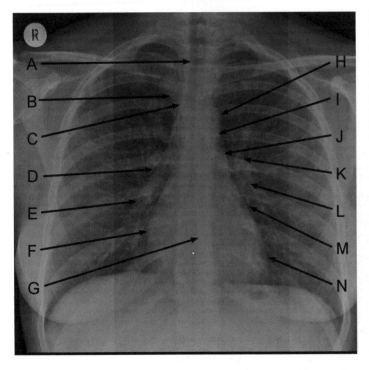

Figure 2.1. This is a normal CXR with mediastinal anatomy labelled.

A, trachea; B, superior vena cava; C, right paratracheal stripe; D, right hilar point; E, right basal pulmonary artery; F, right atrial border; G, azygo–oesophageal line; H, aortic knuckle; I, aorto–pulmonary window; J, pulmonary outflow tract; K, left hilar point; L, left basal pulmonary artery; M, left atrial appendage; N, left ventricular border.

2.2 Lateral CXR

The anatomy of the lateral CXR is arguably harder to interpret than that of the frontal CXR with the hila and hemi-diaphragms overlapping. Usually the lateral is considered in combination with a frontal CXR, but it is important to be aware of where the relevant structures are in order to accurately place any abnormality. *Figure 2.2* explains the basic anatomy of the lateral CXR.

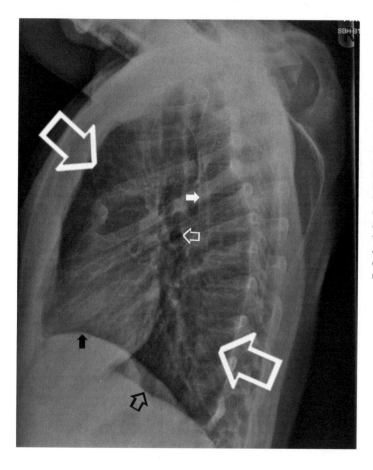

Figure 2.2. This is a lateral CXR of an adult.

Note the difference in the hemi-diaphragms; the right hemi-diaphragm is seen to its anterior extent (black arrow), but the heart obscures the left hemi-diaphragm (open black arrow) in its anterior section. The main areas of interest on a lateral CXR are the retrocardiac and, in particular, the retrosternal regions (large open white arrows) not easily seen on a frontal CXR. Do not confuse the scapulae seen end-on as representing pathology (white arrow); the airway seen end-on at the hilum is the left main bronchus which follows a more horizontal course than the right main bronchus. The trachea can be seen running vertically in the middle of the upper part of the lateral CXR. The aorta is not as clear as you might expect because on the lateral view it is the anterior and posterior walls of the aorta that are projected and for the majority of its course these are adjacent to soft tissue or fat and not aerated lung.

2.3 Normal variants

The following sections describe a range of normal variants that may be seen on CXRs.

2.3.1 Azygos fissure

The azygos fissure (*Fig. 2.3*) is formed when the migration of the azygos vein during fetal development drags four layers of pleura toward the SVC. The fissure is usually incomplete (*Fig. 2.4a*), leaving the segment of lung delineated by the fissure in continuity with the remaining lung, but when complete (*Fig. 2.4b*) an azygos lobe is formed that has its own bronchial supply.

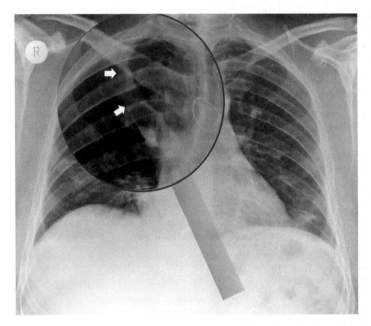

Figure 2.3 Azygos fissure.

The azygos fissure is marked within the magnified area (white arrows).

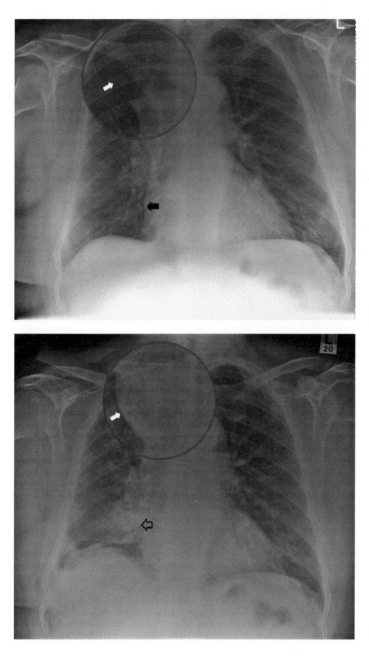

Figure 2.4. Frontal CXRs on a patient with an azygos fissure.

(a) The azygos fissure (white arrow) forms an azygos lobe. Note that in (b) the azygos lobe is consolidated, and consolidation is also present in the right middle lobe obscuring the right heart border (black arrow).

(a)

(b)

2.3.2 Right-sided aortic arch

Although a right-sided aortic arch (*Fig. 2.5*) is classically associated with Tetralogy of Fallot, the finding, along with a double aortic arch, is usually not associated with an underlying cardiac abnormality.

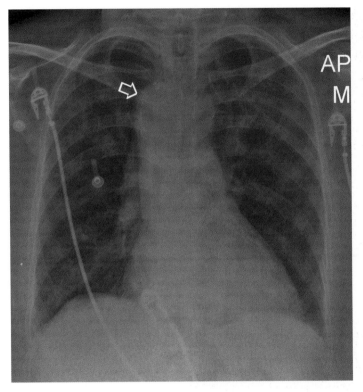

Figure 2.5. Frontal CXR of a patient with a right-sided aortic arch.

The right-sided aortic arch is shown by the open white arrow. Note the extra density on the right of the superior mediastinum and absence of an aorto–pulmonary window on the left.

2.3.3 Dextrocardia

Dextrocardia (*Fig. 2.6*) may be an isolated normal variant but, in association with *situs invertus*, usually indicates the presence of Kartagener's syndrome (*Fig. 2.7*); this is associated with ciliary dysfunction and is classically accompanied by bronchiectasis.

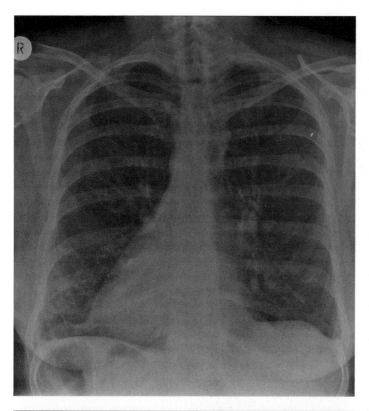

Figure 2.6. Frontal CXR of an adult with dextrocardia and a right-sided aortic arch.

There is no *situs invertus;* the gas shadows under the right hemi-diaphragm are due to the hepatic flexure of the colon.

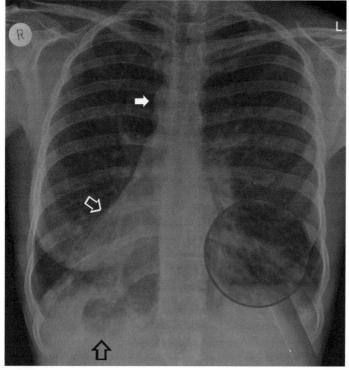

Figure 2.7. CXR of Kartagener's syndrome.

The patient has dextrocardia (open white arrow), right-sided aortic arch (white arrow) and *situs invertus,* with the gastric air bubble appearing on the right (open black arrow). The magnified area demonstrates bronchiectasis.

2.3.4 Bifid rib

Rib abnormalities are often overlooked as one's natural instinct is to ignore the ribs so that the lungs can be interpreted; one way of avoiding this is to turn the CXR through 90° (see *Section 4.5*). *Figure 2.8* shows an example of a bifid rib, of no pathological significance.

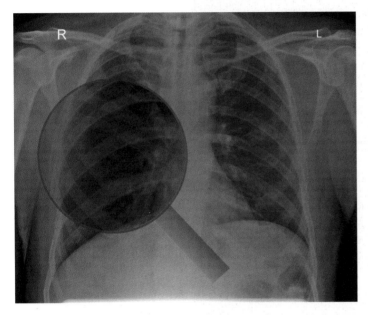

Figure 2.8. Bifid rib.

Note the bifid rib in the magnified area.

2.3.5 Cervical rib

Cervical ribs *(see Fig. 2.9)* can be distinguished from hypoplastic first ribs as they arise from the C7 vertebral body, the transverse processes of which point downwards as opposed to those of the T1 vertebral body that point upwards.

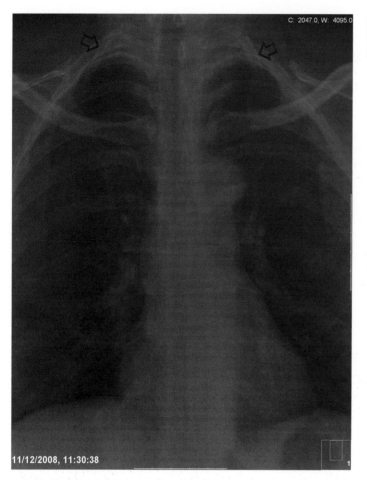

C: 2047.0, W: 4095.0

11/12/2008, 11:30:38

Figure 2.9. Cervical ribs.

Frontal CXR demonstrating bilateral cervical ribs (open black arrows).

03 In-built errors of interpretation

3.1 The eye–brain apparatus

It would be foolish to assume that our eyes pass on to our brains, and subsequently to our consciousness, a true representation of what is being viewed. Eyes do not function like digital cameras, they manufacture an image from basic shapes, contrast interfaces and colours. The fovea is the only area of the retina that can distinguish colour and that only represents a small fraction of our total visual field, yet we perceive colour throughout our visual field and not just at the centre. Because the eye–brain apparatus makes a best guess as to the true picture, it is vulnerable to errors. The adaptive capacity of the eye to generate

a useable image in widely varying ambient lighting levels is remarkable and only possible because the eye is a relative sensor of brightness and cannot determine absolute values. The brightness of an object is determined by the relative brightness of adjacent objects and can therefore appear to change; as a result the eye is easily fooled by interfaces between areas of different brightness. When perceiving a global difference in density on any X-ray, identify the interface between them and obscure it to give a truer representation of the image (*Fig. 3.1*).

(a)

(b)

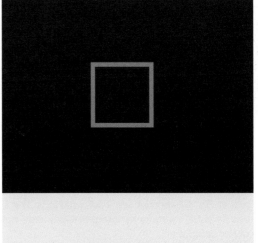

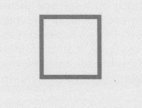

Figure 3.1. Effects of contrast.

(a) The shades of grey to each side are the same. From the left there is a gradient of increasing brightness and from the right a gradient of increasing darkness, the two gradients meet at an interface. The eye is more interested in contrast than absolute brightness levels so makes an assumption about the shades of grey to each side based upon the interface between them. As a result the grey on the left looks lighter than the grey on the right – place a piece of paper over the middle section and the effect is lost.

(b) The squares are actually identical but the difference in the shading of the background gives the impression of a difference in the shading of the square. The square on the darker background appears lighter and that on the darker background lighter.

These effects are outside our conscious control and result from 'bottom up' processing. A more alarming deficiency results from 'top down' processing, where a preconception about how an image should look results in an inability to see the image as it is. Look at *Figure 3.2* and you should see a collection of shapes of differing shades of grey.

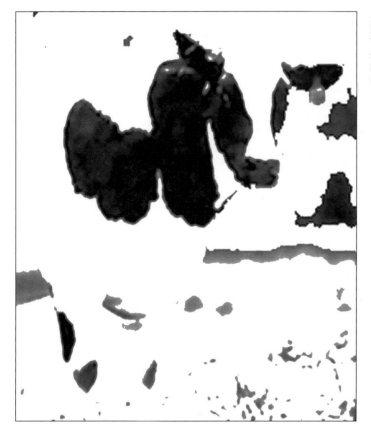

Figure 3.2. What is this an image of?

The answer is in the *Appendix*, but don't look too soon as when you know what this is you will not be able to look at this picture again and fail to see it for what it is.

Having seen the answer in the *Appendix*, I challenge you to look back at *Fig. 3.2* and not see it for what it is. The brain automatically uses its visual memory to interpret the image before you have any conscious input.

When viewing an X-ray one should always be aware of the uncontrollable errors of visual perception, and an effort should be made to view the image systematically to avoid a reliance on a generic overview of the image. If areas of different density / brightness are perceived, it is worthwhile obscuring the interface between two such areas to ensure there is a real difference in density.

3.2 The snapshot

When viewing any CXR, a snapshot impression is made by the viewer in deciding whether the CXR is normal or abnormal.

3.2.1 Snapshot decision 'normal'

Once the viewer has decided the CXR is normal, any abnormality on that CXR will become very difficult to see because from then on the viewer has a preconceived notion about the CXR and, even more alarmingly, has probably perceived and discarded the abnormality in that first snapshot impression. This explains the times when, despite staring at an X-ray, a viewer fails to see an abnormality until it is pointed out to them, and then they cannot understand how they missed something so obvious.

3.2.2 Snapshot decision 'abnormal'

The danger inherent in detecting an abnormality immediately is that of satisfaction of search (SOS); SOS describes the tendency to stop looking for abnormalities when one has already been found (see *Section 3.4*).

3.3 Image misinterpretation

The brain is keen to see images that are familiar to it, which is why we see recognisable objects in the clouds. Overlapping structures on a CXR are readily interpreted as parts of a single recognisable structure such as a cavity or a nodule, or even a mass (see *Fig. 3.3*). On seeing what appears to be a cavity or nodule, try determining what lines on the X-ray are giving you that impression; are they actually just overlapping structures?

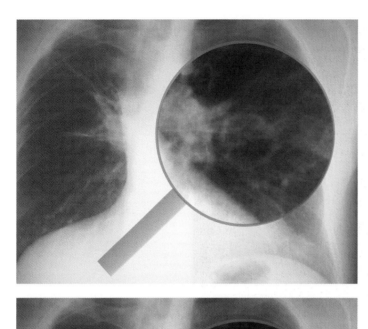

(a)

(b)

Figure 3.3. Cavity?

The magnified area is in the region of the left hilum where appearances suggest a thick-walled cavity (a). The broken lines (b) mark the margins of two vessels that are creating the illusion of a cavity.

3.4 Satisfaction of search

Satisfaction of search (SOS) is a basic error of human nature that must be actively opposed. The principle is that on finding an abnormality you are unlikely to search for, or find, a second abnormality. This, in combination with the snapshot impression described earlier, can conceal quite obvious abnormalities from you. Now take a look at the following CXRs (*Figs 3.4, 3.5* and *3.6*).

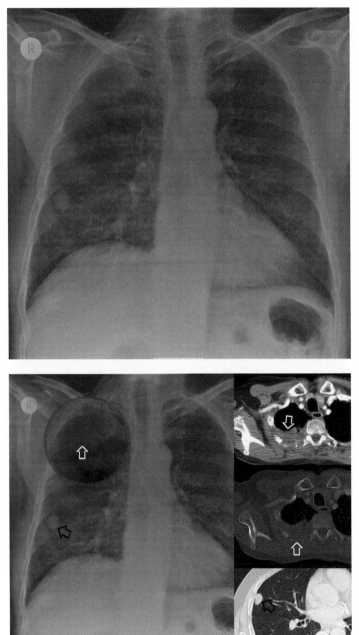

Figure 3.4. SOS 1.

Have you spotted the nodule in the right lower zone? Try turning the image through 90 degrees. Now look at *Figure 4.6.*

Figure 3.5. SOS 2.

You should have seen the nodule (open black arrow) and probably, given that the subject of this section is satisfaction of search, noticed the increased density in the apex, but did you spot the rib destruction (open white arrow)?

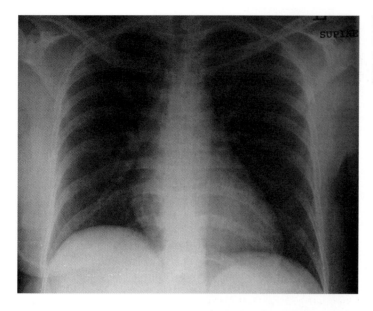

Figure 3.6. SOS 3.

Frontal CXR of an adult female in whom there is a discrepancy in the density of the lower zones. Can you identify the abnormalities? The answer is in *Section 3.5*.

3.5 Ignoring the ribs

The ribs are usually considered an irritant on X-rays, causing apparent abnormalities that distract from the interpretation of the lungs; as a result one becomes quite adept at ignoring the ribs automatically. Unfortunately, this means that rib-based abnormalities, as in *Figure 3.6*, are readily overlooked. One way to avoid this is to change the orientation of the CXR; if you turn the CXR through 90° you are forced to interpret an image that no longer looks like a routine CXR, giving you the opportunity to interpret the ribs as an entity in themselves (see *Fig. 3.7*). In the examples in *Section 3.4*, did you find that turning the CXR through 90° helped you to identify the rib abnormalities? In *Fig. 3.6*, the subject has had a mastectomy for breast cancer, and the eighth rib has been destroyed by a metastasis.

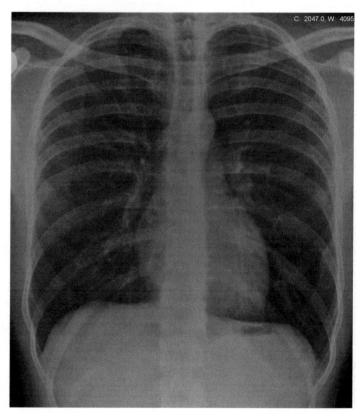

Figure 3.7. Rib abnormality.

Try rotating the CXR through 90° to help identify the abnormality. The answer is given in the *Appendix*.

04 The fundamentals of CXR interpretation

4.1 The silhouette sign

A silhouette is the outline of an object defined by the shadow it casts. In terms of a CXR, the silhouette sign is based on the same concept except that X-rays, to which soft tissues are translucent rather than opaque, replace light. The formation of a silhouette on a CXR depends on two tissues of sufficiently different density lying against each other in such a way that two adjacent X-rays will pass through one, or the other, but not both tissues. In this way, when the adjacent X-rays reach the film / detector they will generate different shades of grey, which, if sufficiently different will be discernable (see *Fig. 4.1*). This is the principle that underlies all plain X-rays, but in the chest it is particularly important as aerated lung, which absorbs hardly any X-rays, generates excellent silhouettes (*Fig. 4.1*). Unfortunately, the contrast resolution of plain radiography is such that silhouettes are only formed by bone, soft tissue, fat and aerated lung. Note that vessels, lymph nodes, muscle, fluid, and connective tissue are all of soft tissue density and are therefore of the same density on plain X-rays (*Fig. 4.2*).

The loss of the normal silhouettes on a CXR results from an increase in density of the adjacent lower density tissue; on a CXR this is usually aerated lung adjacent to a soft tissue structure, indicating a pathological process. Knowing the anatomy of the silhouettes not only allows the recognition of pathology but also aids localisation of that pathology.

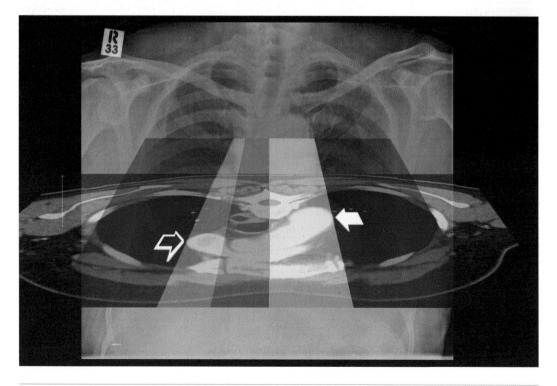

Figure 4.1. Silhouette CXR.

The axial CT image at the level of the aortic arch is projected in perspective over a CXR and the shaded lines match the air–soft tissue interfaces to the silhouettes they form.

21

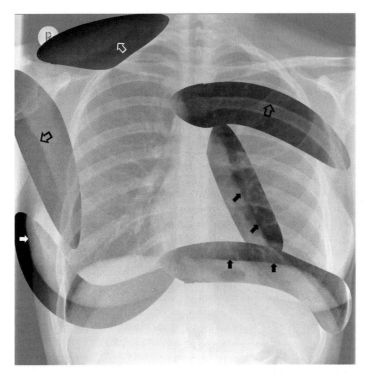

Figure 4.2. Interfaces.

This is a normal CXR with a few areas highlighted and magnified to demonstrate examples of the various soft tissue interfaces visible on a CXR:

- soft tissue / aerated lung – solid black arrows
- soft tissue / air – solid white arrow (contour of the breast)
- soft tissue / bone – open black arrow
- soft tissue / fat – open white arrow

Another reason for not seeing an interface between two tissues of sufficiently different density on CXR is because the orientation of the interface is not in line with the incident X-rays (*Fig. 4.3*).

Perhaps the most important silhouettes on the CXR tend not to be described as such. The density of blood-filled vessels is not great, but is sufficiently different to aerated lung to render all but the very peripheral vessels visible. Indeed, when the bronchi become too small to be seen and the normal lung interstitium is too fine to be seen, the vessels are the only indication of the presence of lung for the majority of the CXR. As a result, it is the appearance of the vessels that gives the most immediate indication of lung pathology.

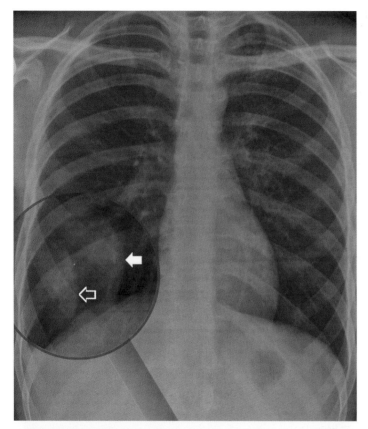

(a)

Figure 4.3. Pleural based lesions on CXR and CT.

These are the (a) CXR and (b) CT images of two pleural based lesions. Due to the curvature of the chest wall only the medial margins of the lesions cast a silhouette (arrows); the remainder of the margins are in the wrong orientation to form a silhouette.

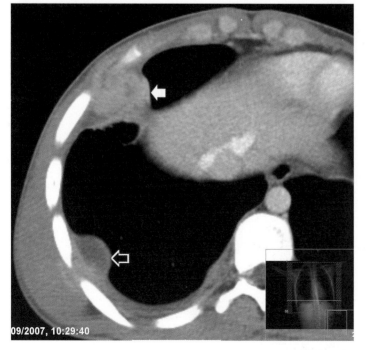

(b)

4.2 Suggested scheme for CXR viewing

The following scheme suggests a systematic way of viewing a CXR that is not determined by anatomical boundaries. If you develop your own scheme bear in mind the potential pitfalls detailed here.

1. Check the name and date of the film.
2. Is the film the correct way round (side marker)?
3. Is the film PA or AP (assume PA if no alternative indicated on the CXR)?
4. Is the subject erect, semi-erect or supine (AP erect is, in reality, semi-erect)?

Begin in the top left-hand corner of the film (patient's right shoulder) and then use the following systematic scanning approach:

A. Scan from left to right and back again *(Fig. 4.4)*.
B. Scan from top left to bottom left *(Fig. 4.5)*.
C. Move to under the right diaphragm and scan up to the right apex *(Fig. 4.6)*.
D. From the right apex scan down the right mediastinal contour *(Fig. 4.7)*.
E. Scan up the centre of the film *(Fig. 4.8)*.
F. Scan down the left mediastinal contour *(Fig. 4.9)*.
G. Move to under the left hemi-diaphragm (the gastric fundus and the spleen reside here) and scan up to the left apex *(Fig. 4.10)*.
H. Move to the left shoulder and scan down the left periphery of the chest *(Fig. 4.11)*.
I. Finally compare the lung parenchyma left to right in the upper, mid and lower zones *(Fig. 4.12)*.

This scheme is easy to follow and encourages interpretation of the CXR unhindered by the bias created by a snapshot impression.

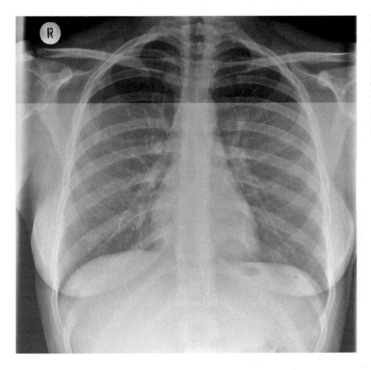

Figure 4.4. Scan from left to right and back again.

Check the soft tissues and bones of the shoulder girdle (clavicles, scapulae) and neck; are there any bony lesions (fractures, deposits, cervical ribs, joint abnormalities, etc.) or soft tissue masses? Is the trachea normal (position, calibre)? Compare the apices of the lung: are they the same density? Return to the top left-hand corner repeating the above observations.

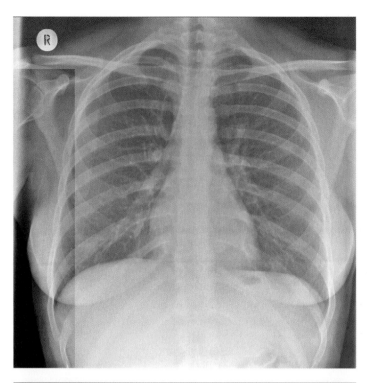

Figure 4.5. Scan from top left to bottom left.

Check the soft tissues of the chest wall, the lateral aspect of the ribs, the peripheral lung, pleura and costophrenic angle.

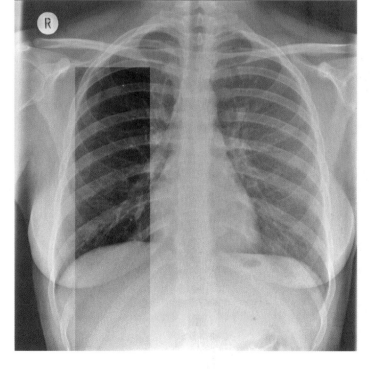

Figure 4.6. Move to under the right diaphragm and scan up to the right apex.

Check behind the diaphragm as there is enough space here to 'hide' a 7–8 cm tumour. Observe the parenchyma of the right lung: are the vessels visible and of normal calibre? If the vessels are obscured that suggests abnormal opacity in the adjacent lung.

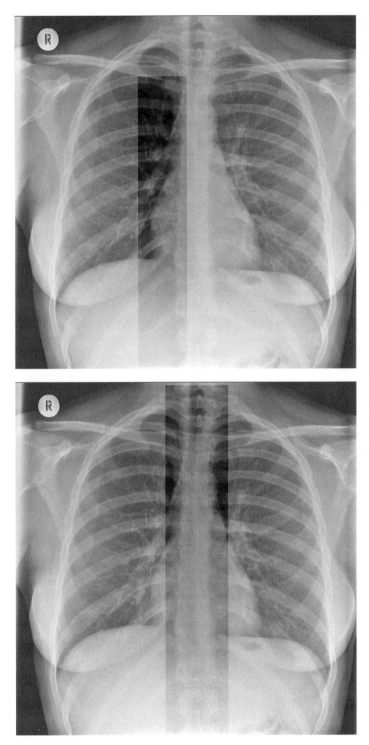

Figure 4.7. From the right apex scan down the right mediastinal contour.

The right paratracheal stripe should be visible. Is the mediastinal contour visible? Check the position of the hilar point: this should be at the level of the lateral extent of the right 6th rib. End at the right cardiophrenic angle, which is where the inferior vena cava lies.

Figure 4.8. Scan up the centre of the film.

Note the structures that should be visible behind the heart, particularly the spine, paraspinal region and azygo-oesophageal line (often overlooked). Is the mediastinum central, the carina normal, and the trachea normal in position and calibre?

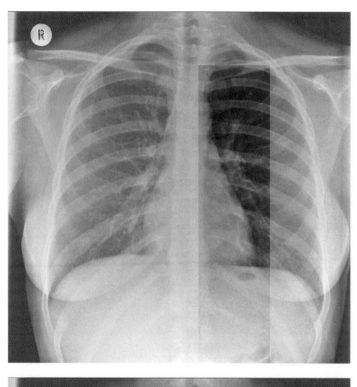

Figure 4.9. Scan down the left mediastinal contour.

Check the aortic knuckle, aorto–pulmonary window, the left hilar point (1–1.5 cm higher than the right hilar point), and the left contour of the heart (pulmonary outflow tract, left atrial appendage and left ventricle). End at the left cardiophrenic angle.

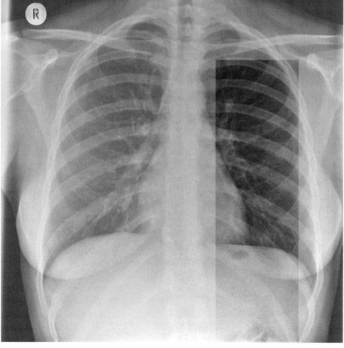

Figure 4.10. Move to under the left hemi-diaphragm, and scan up to the left apex.

Scan up the film looking at the lung parenchyma ending in the left apex. Under the diaphragm are the gastric fundus and the spleen.

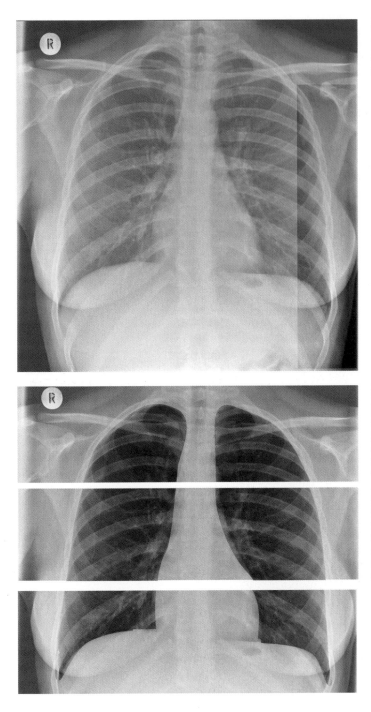

Figure 4.11. Scan from the left shoulder, scan down the left periphery of the chest.

Concentrate on the peripheral lung, ribs and soft tissues of the chest wall.

Figure 4.12. Compare the lung parenchyma left to right in the upper, mid and lower zones.

Comparison of the two lung fields can be performed by switching your gaze from one to the other rapidly, but this relies on immediate visual memory and is susceptible to the errors outlined in the section on the eye–brain apparatus (see *Section 3.1*). By developing a technique whereby you centre your gaze on the mediastinum, but concentrate your perception on both lungs simultaneously, you are utilizing the area of your retina surrounding the fovea; this area contains the greatest density of rods designed to detect contrast differences which are ideal for this type of comparison. Colour perception is irrelevant when viewing a plain film.

4.3 Review areas

In the 'busy' or obscured areas of the CXR an abnormality can easily be missed; these areas warrant a second look and are termed review areas (see *Fig. 4.13*). In the following section the various review areas are highlighted and the typical abnormalities and structures potentially hidden in these areas are demonstrated.

4.3.1 The apices

The apices of the lung are obscured by overlying first rib and clavicle causing an increase in the density of the area at the expense of clarity in the low density aerated lung. In addition, at the extreme apex it is not unusual to have a 'cap' of pleural thickening that is of no clinical significance.

The best way to approach the apices is by comparing the density of the two sides; if there is a difference in opacity, can this be explained by the overlying ribs?

If a parenchymal abnormality is suspected, in the first instance a lordotic view should be performed whereby the angle of the incident X-rays is altered; for a PA film the X-rays are angled downwards and for an AP film upwards (see *Figs 4.14* and *4.15*).

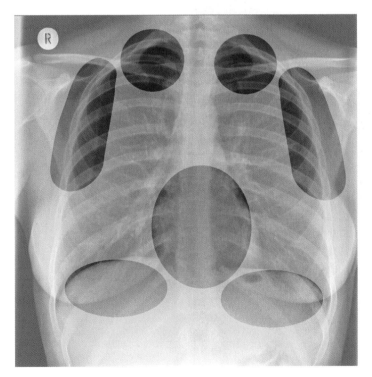

Figure 4.13. Review areas.

This image highlights the areas of the CXR that should be revisited as abnormalities are easily missed in these areas.

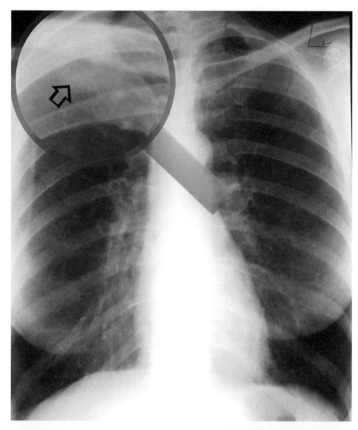

Figure 4.14. (a) Standard PA film and (b) lordotic view.

The magnified area on this PA film (a) raises the possibility of a cavitating lesion in the right apex (open black arrow). The index of suspicion is low as there are numerous overlapping structures in this region so CT scanning would seem to be over-zealous. On the lordotic view (b) the relevant area of lung is confirmed as clear.

(a)

(b)

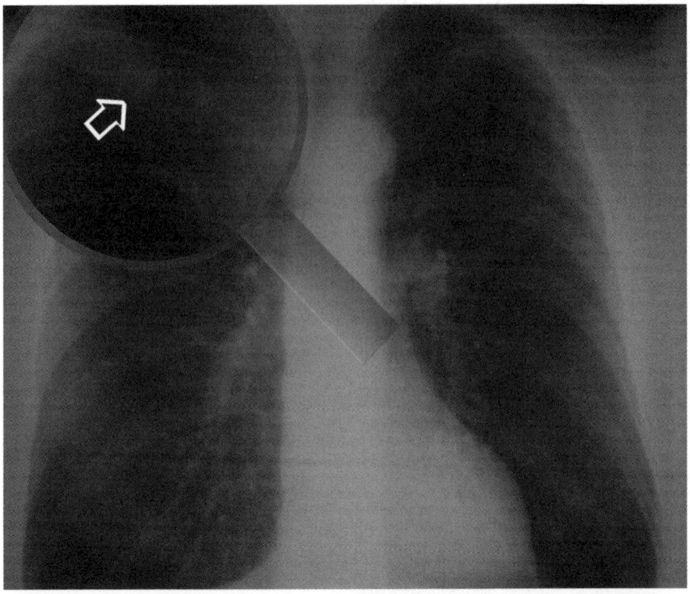

Figure 4.15. (a) Standard PA film and (b) lordotic view. The initial PA CXR (a) demonstrates subtle differences between the two apices; the open white arrow in the magnified region highlights a possible lung parenchymal lesion. A subsequent lordotic view (b) projects the first rib and clavicle cranially leaving the lesion readily identifiable.

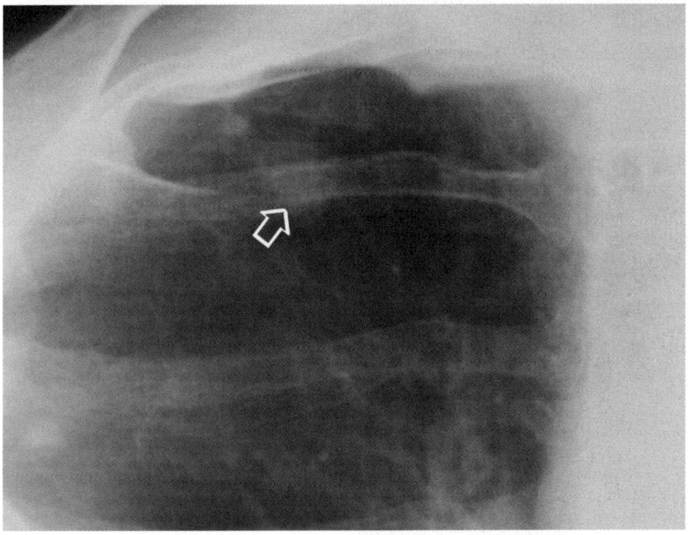

(a)

(b)

4.3.2 The thoracic inlet

The only structure readily seen at the thoracic inlet is the trachea as it contains air; the oesophagus may be visualized, but air found that high up in the oesophagus would normally only be a transient finding. Most of the vessels in the superior mediastinum are not readily seen, because the interfaces between them and the aerated lung in the apices are at the wrong orientation to be seen on a frontal CXR (*Fig. 4.16*); the SVC in particular, and sometimes the left subclavian artery, are only discernable below the sternal notch (*Fig. 4.17*).

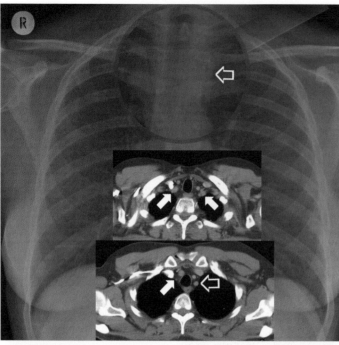

Figure 4.16. Thoracic inlet.

This is a normal CXR with the thoracic inlet magnified. Note that the left subclavian artery may form a silhouette (open white arrow), but the other superior mediastinal contours, particularly above the sternal notch, are at the wrong orientation to form a silhouette on a frontal chest radiograph (white arrows).

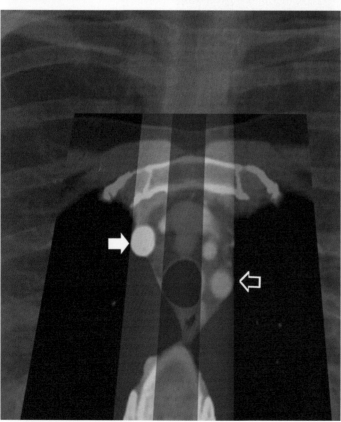

Figure 4.17. Arch vessels.

Limited view of the upper mediastinum with a projection of part of an axial CT scan at that level. The shading identifies the interfaces between aerated lung and the SVC (white arrow) and left subclavian artery (open white arrow); the margins of the trachea are also shaded.

The trachea may be narrowed due to intrinsic disease or external compression, or deviated due to an external mass (most commonly a goitre; *Figs 4.18* and *4.19*). Note that only the coronal diameter is appreciated on a frontal CXR and that a significant compression in the sagittal plane, as may be caused by a retrosternal goitre, can only be seen on a lateral view of the thoracic inlet. Care should be taken not to confuse the false cords as pathological tracheal stenosis; false cords represent a normal narrowing of the trachea just inferior to the larynx that is often visible during the valsalva manoeuvre, encouraged by the command 'breathe in and hold your breath' (see *Fig. 4.20*).

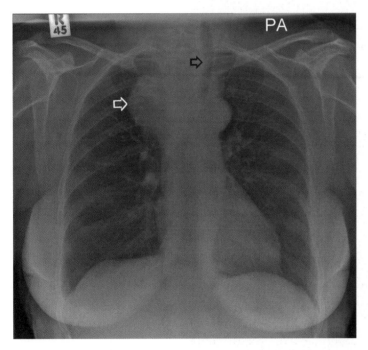

Figure 4.18. Goitre.

Frontal CXR of an adult female with a goitre. Note the deviation of the trachea (open black arrow) and the lateral margin of the enlarged thyroid causing a silhouette with adjacent aerated lung (open white arrow).

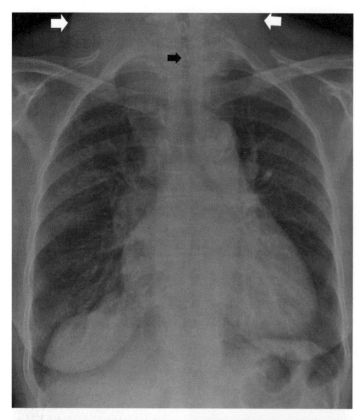

Figure 4.19. Large goitre.

Frontal CXR of an adult with a very large goitre, the lateral margins of which are seen (white arrows). This goitre encases the trachea and therefore causes narrowing (black arrow) rather than deviation.

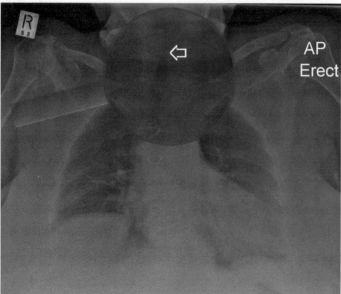

Figure 4.20. False cords.

This is an AP portable CXR. Note the narrowing of the trachea in the magnified area (open white arrow); this is the false cords and should not be confused with pathology.

4.3.3 Overlying the scapulae

Ideally the scapulae should be projected off the chest but this is often not the case. As a result, the upper lateral regions of the lung on a CXR are of increased density due to superimposed scapulae. As you become familiar with viewing CXRs you will expect some increased opacity in this region and therefore a subtle real abnormality such as a soft tissue nodule unrelated to the scapulae can easily be overlooked (*Fig. 4.21*).

4.3.4 Costophrenic angles

The costophrenic angle should be 'sharp', i.e. the diaphragm should form an acute angle with the chest wall. 'Blunting' of the costophrenic angle indicates that there is soft tissue or fluid where the lowest limits of the lung should be; this is usually due to pleural fluid or thickening (*Fig. 4.22*). Caution should be taken when the lungs are of large volume causing flattening of the hemi-diaphragms; in such cases blunting of the costophrenic angles may be due to the diaphragmatic slips becoming visible, because the normally quite deep lateral pleural recess is exposed by over-expanded lung (*Fig. 4.23*).

The area of lung seen at the costophrenic angle is the most peripheral gravity-dependent region. In circumstances where excess fluid is accumulating in the lung it tends to accumulate between the secondary pulmonary lobules. The secondary pulmonary lobule is a defined unit of lung that is polygonal in shape and each is supplied by its own respiratory bronchiole. The lung consists of many such lobules of varying size fitted together like a 3-D jigsaw. Where these lobules contact each other is termed the interlobular septum. These septa are not usually visible on a CXR, but if they become thickened due to accumulation of fluid (e.g. in left heart failure, or lymphangitis carcinomatosa) they may be seen, but only when in the correct orientation to the incident X-ray (*Fig. 4.24*). These thickened septal lines are best appreciated at the costophrenic angles where there are numerous septa in line with the X-ray beam but no normal vascular structures visible to obscure them.

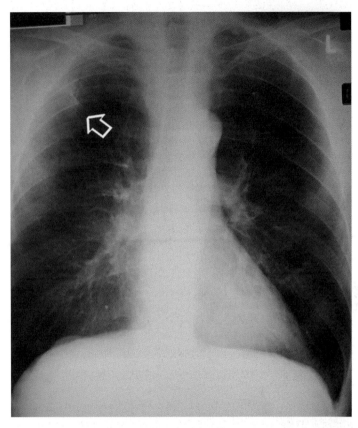

Figure 4.21. Overlying scapula.

This frontal CXR demonstrates a soft tissue nodule (open white arrow), projected over the medial border of the right scapula, that could easily be overlooked.

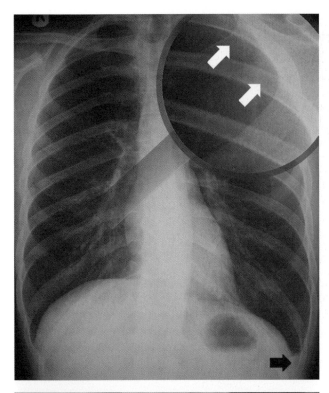

Figure 4.22. Subtle pneumothorax.

This is the frontal CXR of a young man with a spontaneous pneumothorax. Note the blunting of the left costophrenic angle (black arrow) due to the accumulation of the pleural fluid at the base rather than being normally distributed over the surface of the lung. The lung edge can be discerned by careful scrutiny (white arrows). In the context of sudden onset chest pain, with a unilateral blunting of the costophrenic angle, a spontaneous pneumothorax should be excluded.

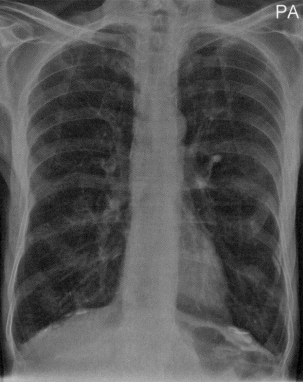

Figure 4.23. COPD.

This is the frontal CXR of a patient with chronic airway disease. Due to the over-expansion of the lungs, the diaphragms are flattened and the diaphragmatic slips give the appearance of small bilateral effusions. There are also bilateral calcified plaques in this patient indicating a previous exposure to asbestos.

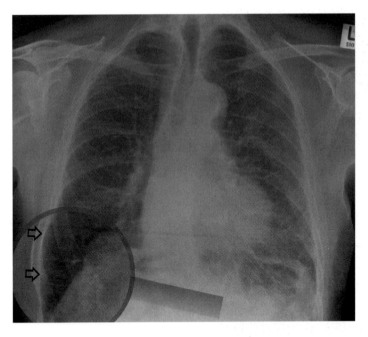

Figure 4.24. Septal lines at the costophrenic angle. Frontal CXR of a patient in left heart failure. In the magnified area note the horizontal lines (open black arrows) extending from the pleural surface: these are septal or 'Kerley B' lines.

4.3.5 Under the hemi-diaphragms

A large amount of aerated lung is projected behind the hemi-diaphragms which tend to peak anteriorly; note the margin of the hemi-diaphragm giving rise to the diaphragmatic silhouette also lies anterior to the midline (see *Fig. 2.2*). High kV and, in particular, digital CXRs display a significant amount of this 'hidden' lung tissue and these areas are worth a second look as review areas.

Lucency beneath the hemi-diaphragms indicates gas, either free or in the bowel. Gas in the bowel outlines the inner wall of the intestines and usually has curved margins in keeping with the internal contour of tubular structures. On the left the fundus of the stomach and sometimes the splenic flexure of the colon lie beneath the hemi-diaphragm. On the right the liver usually occupies the sub-diaphragmatic space, but in some individuals there is interposition of the hepatic flexure of the colon so that gas under the right hemi-diaphragm may still be a normal finding. Free gas lies between the normal abdominal viscera of the abdomen and tends to form sharp margins (*Figs 4.25* and *4.26*).

If the CXR findings are uncertain, then a lateral decubitus AXR view should resolve the issue; the free gas will travel to the least dependent area, i.e. the upper most lateral margin of the abdomen, and it is readily appreciated there. Similarly, a supine CXR will fail to identify free sub-diaphragmatic gas because the free gas will accumulate under the anterior abdominal wall.

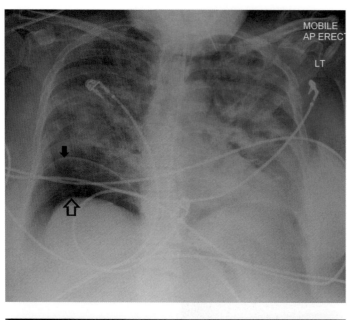

Figure 4.25. Free gas showing on AP film.

AP CXR of an adult with diffuse metastatic breast cancer as the cause for the diffuse bilateral patchy opacities. Note the right hemi-diaphragm (black arrow) is separated from the liver surface (open black arrow) by free intra-peritoneal gas from a perforated bowel.

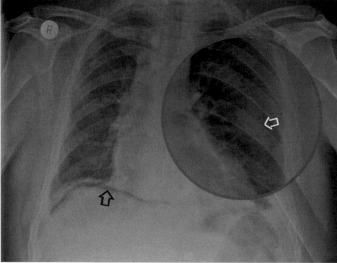

Figure 4.26. Gas under hemi-diaphragm pseudopneumothorax.

AP CXR of an adult. There is free gas under the right hemi-diaphragm, due to a perforation, that extends medially to the spine, excluding atelectasis as a cause for the appearances. Note that in the magnified area there is a line that mimics a lung edge, but this is actually due to a skin fold.

4.3.6 Behind the heart

Thoracic spine

On a well taken CXR the thoracic spine should be visible, superimposed on the mediastinal shadow. On a CXR where the spine is not visible the exposure is insufficient and the CXR should be viewed with caution because a significant portion of the thorax has not been adequately visualized.

Vertebral height and alignment of the thoracic spine may be appreciated on a CXR, particularly end plate changes (*Fig. 4.27*), scoliosis (see *Fig. 6.2*), even ankylosis (*Fig. 4.28*). Loss of vertebral height in the mid and upper thoracic spine may be difficult to detect as the thoracic spine is kyphotic and therefore most of the vertebral bodies in this part of the thoracic spine are not in line with the X-rays. Nevertheless, vertebral height in the lower thoracic spine, behind the heart, may be determined and should not be ignored.

A clue to spinal pathology may be the presence of extra paraspinal soft tissue, either haematoma secondary to trauma, or as a result of an infectious or neoplastic process (*Fig. 4.29*).

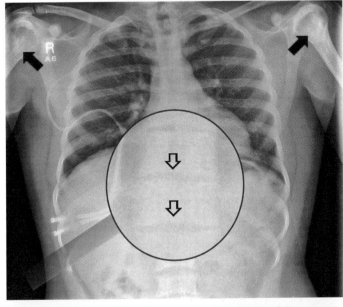

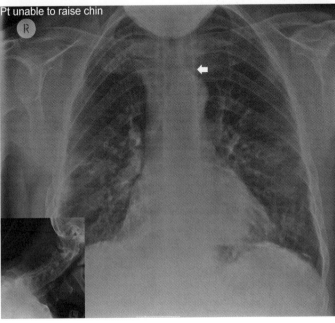

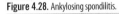

Figure 4.27. Sickle cell disease.

Frontal CXR of a patient with sickle cell disease. Note in the magnified area the vertebral end plate depression (open black arrows). Bony sclerosis, most notable in the humeral heads (black arrows), is due to the sickle cell disease.

Figure 4.28. Ankylosing spondilitis.

Frontal CXR of an adult with ankylosing spondilitis. Note the ossification of the paraspinal ligaments (white arrow) and the ankylosis of the cervical spine (shown in the inset picture) explaining why this patient could not raise his chin.

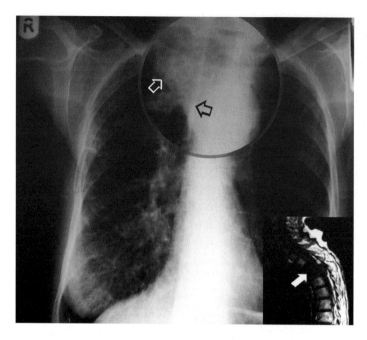

Figure 4.29. Spinal metastases.

Frontal CXR on a patient with metastatic cancer. There are metastases in the upper thoracic spine best seen on the MRI insert (white arrow) causing paraspinal soft tissue density on the CXR (open white arrow) Note the preservation of the right para-tracheal stripe indicating that the abnormality lies posteriorly.

Descending aorta

The lateral contour of the descending aorta is adjacent to aerated lung and therefore can be seen projected behind the heart, but the medial border is not appreciated on CXR (*Fig. 4.30*), and therefore the calibre of the descending aorta is not readily appreciated unless markedly abnormal (*Fig. 4.31*). A tortuous descending aorta is a far more common cause of a deviated lateral margin of the descending aorta than an aneurysm (*Fig. 4.32*).

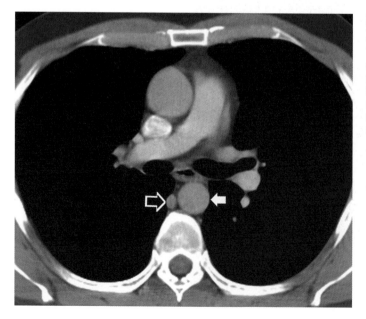

Figure 4.30. Descending aorta.

CT images just below the level of the carina. The left margin of the descending aorta (white arrow) is adjacent to aerated lung and generates a silhouette. The right side of the descending aorta is not adjacent to aerated lung; the silhouette seen on the CXR is actually due to the azygos vein and is not a reliable indicator of the position of the medial margin of the descending aorta.

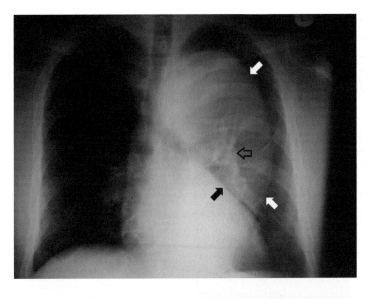

Figure 4.31. Descending aortic aneurysm.

Frontal CXR demonstrating a large descending aortic aneurysm; note that the preservation of the left heart border and hilar point localize this soft tissue to the posterior chest. The contour of the descending aorta is markedly displaced (white arrows); a clue to this being aneurysmal rather than unfolding is the increase in diameter of the arch.

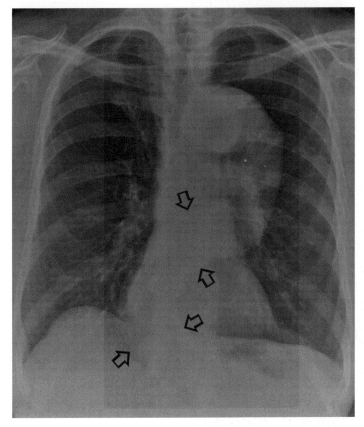

Figure 4.32. Unfolded aorta.

Frontal CXR demonstrating an unfolded aorta. Some of the margins of this are marked (open black arrows). Note that, unlike the aneurysm in *Fig. 4.31*, the left contour of the descending aorta remains close enough to the likely position of the right margin of the aorta to retain a more normal calibre. Also, the lateral contour of the aorta does not extend upwards from the arch as it did with the aneurysm in *Fig. 4.31*.

Oesophagus

The oesophagus is not normally seen on a CXR but may become visible if it contains air (*Fig. 4.33*) or is abnormally dilated as in achalasia (*Fig. 4.34*). When the stomach protrudes into the mediastinum, a hiatus hernia, it occupies a region of the mediastinum usually occupied only by the oesophagus and therefore, even when small, it is likely to abut adjacent aerated lung, forming a line that is visible on a CXR. In addition, there is often air and fluid in the stomach and an air–fluid level may be seen: a horizontal line separating an area of low density above (air) from an area of high density below (fluid), provided the CXR is taken with the patient erect (*Fig. 4.35*). Note that the air–fluid level will only be apparent when the air–fluid interface is in line with the X-ray beam, hence the necessity for the CXR to be erect so that the incident X-rays are horizontal in orientation (see later). Furthermore, if there is solid material in the hiatus hernia there may be no air–fluid level to see (*Fig. 4.36*).

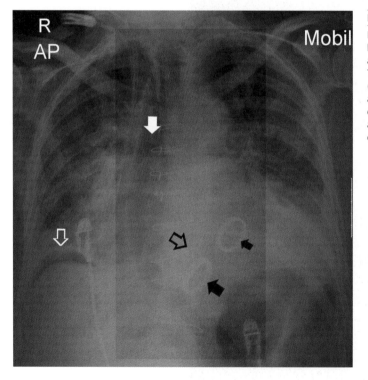

Figure 4.33. Free gas in oesophagus from a burp.

Frontal CXR on a patient that has had mitral (small black arrow), tricuspid (large black arrow) and aortic valve (open black arrow) replacements. The oesophagus is readily identified filled with air (white arrow) but the appearance did not persist as would be expected if the cause was oesophageal dilatation and the patient has probably just burped as the CXR was taken. In addition there is free sub-diaphragmatic gas (open white arrow).

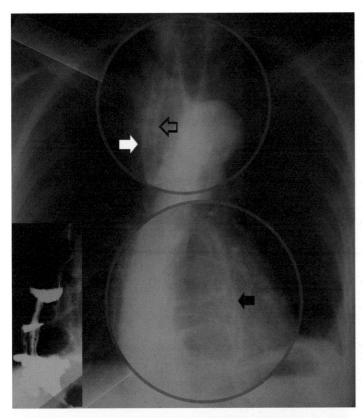

Figure 4.34. Achalasia.

Frontal CXR with a barium swallow insert. Note, in the upper magnified area, the wall of the oesophagus (white arrow) is seen separate to the right tracheal wall (open black arrow). In the lower magnified area the dilated oesophagus is again noted, and the lateral wall is marked by the black arrow. The barium swallow confirms the markedly dilated oesophagus in this case due to achalasia.

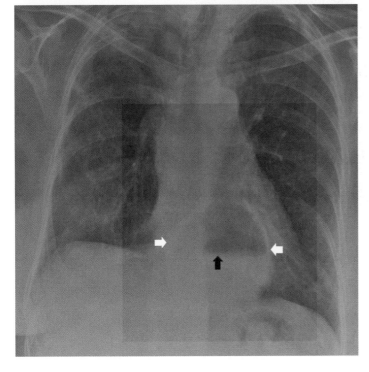

Figure 4.35. Hiatus hernia with air–fluid level shown.

Frontal CXR showing a hiatus hernia. Note the lateral margins of the hernia (white arrows) and the air–fluid level (black arrow).

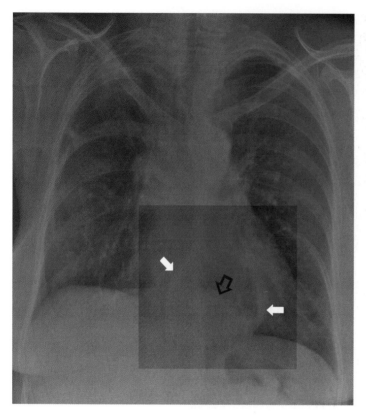

Figure 4.36. Hiatus hernia with food.

Frontal CXR of the same patient as in *Fig. 4.35*. Note the margins of the hiatus hernia (black arrows), but in this case there is no air–fluid level as the hernia contains food (open black arrow).

Azygo-oesophageal line

The azygo-oesophageal line is formed by the interface between the azygos and/or the right side of the oesophagus and adjacent aerated lung (*Fig. 4.37*); it ascends vertically, overlying the vertebral bodies (the spinous processes can cause confusion), and then arches to the patient's right as the azygos vein passes over the right main bronchus to drain into the superior vena cava. The line does not extend above the carina. If the azygo-oesophageal line is seen, and this is not always the case, then bulging or loss of the line indicates sub-carinal pathology, usually lymphadenopathy (*Figs 4.38* and *4.39*).

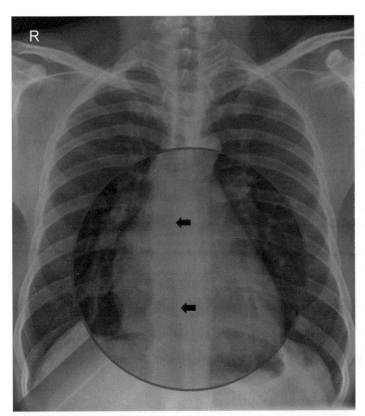

Figure 4.37. Azygo-oesophageal line.

Frontal CXR demonstrating the azygo-oesophageal line (black arrows). The soft tissue / aerated lung interface giving rise to the line is marked on the CT image in *Fig. 4.30*.

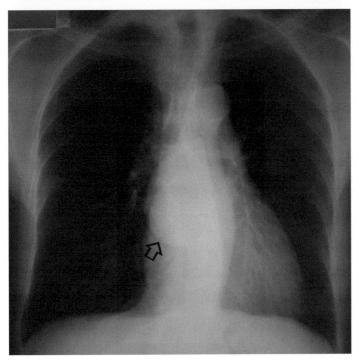

Figure 4.38. Sub-carinal adenopathy.

Frontal CXR showing sub-carinal adenopathy causing bulging of the azygo-oesophageal line (open black arrow).

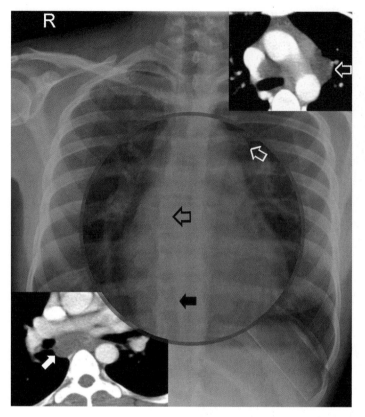

Figure 4.39. Aorto-pulmonary window and sub-carinal adenopathy.

A more subtle example of sub-carinal adenopathy. In this image the azygo-oesophageal line (black arrow) ceases to become visible (open black arrow) due to the sub-carinal adenopathy (lower left inset, white arrow) generating a soft tissue–air interface in the wrong orientation to show up on a frontal CXR. Note there is also an aorto-pulmonary window adenopathy on this CXR (open white arrow and top right inset).

4.3.7 Hidden lung

Approximately 30% of the left lower lobe (LLL) is projected behind the heart; a lesser proportion of the right lower lobe (RLL) is obscured by the heart, but still sufficient to 'hide' sizeable abnormalities (*Fig. 4.40*). In addition there is a significant amount of lung hidden behind the hemi-diaphragms (*Fig. 4.41*). As elsewhere in the chest, the parenchymal vessels are visible, but care must be taken not to overlook any abnormality in this part of the lung; the general increase in density due to the heart reduces the observer's sensitivity for detecting abnormal densities (*Fig. 4.42*). Particular mention must be made of LLL collapse, which is dealt with in detail in *Section 5.1.5*.

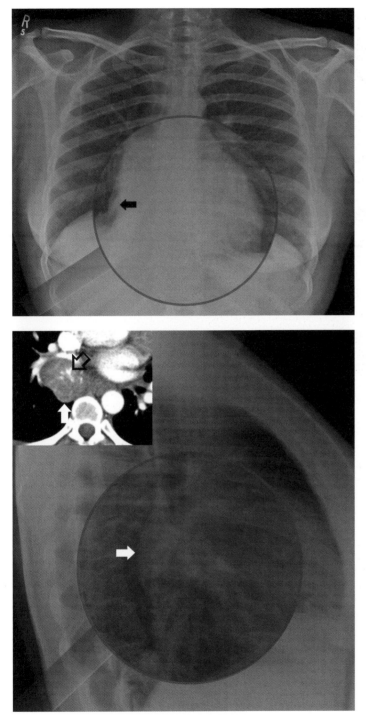

(a)

(b)

Figure 4.40. Carcinoid behind heart CXR.

Frontal (a) and lateral (b) CXRs demonstrating a subtle mass behind the heart. The lateral margin is marked with a black arrow, and the white arrow marks the right heart border. Note the difference in density between the right heart and left heart. On the lateral view (b) and the CT inset, the posterior margin of the carcinoid is marked (white arrow). Note the calcification (open black arrow) often found in carcinoid tumours.

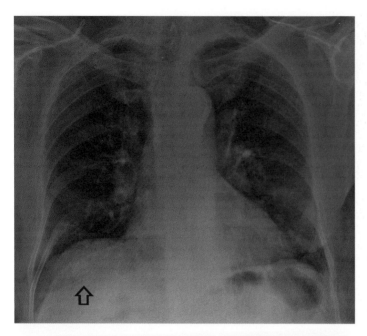

Figure 4.41. Deposit behind diaphragm.

There is a 2.5 cm metastatic deposit behind the right hemi-diaphragm (open black arrow).

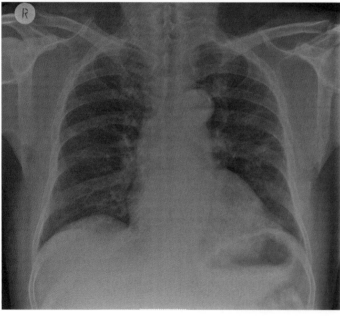

Figure 4.42. Unmarked hidden mass.

Take a look at this CXR. Now you have been sensitized to detecting masses in the hidden areas of the lung, can you identify the 4–5 cm mass on this CXR? The answer is in *Fig. 4.43*.

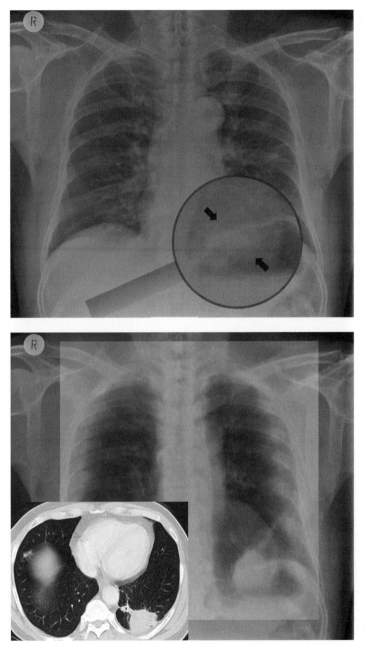

Figure 4.43. (a) Marked hidden mass and (b) same mass shown on a CT with coronal overlay.

This is a tricky one with the heart and left hemi-diaphragm obscuring what is actually a large mass (black arrows). (b) has an inset demonstrating the mass on an axial CT image and there is a coronal overlay to localize the mass on the CXR.

(a)

(b)

4.3.8 The cardiophrenic angles

The cardiophrenic angles form at the point where the heart shadow meets the diaphragms. The angle made by the heart and diaphragms at the cardiophrenic angles is acute in nature but blunted by the cardiac fat pads. As a result, the density in this region is in between aerated lung and soft tissue and can confuse the eye. It gives the impression of an abnormality that doesn't exist by 'blurring' the silhouette of the heart (*Fig. 4.44*), or obscuring a real abnormality as, with experience, the viewer will come to accept a slightly abnormal appearance in this region (*Fig. 4.45*).

When prominent, a fat pad can be difficult to discard unless previous imaging confirms that it is a consistent feature.

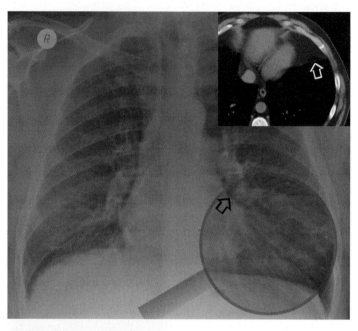

Figure 4.44. Fat pad.

Frontal CXR of an adult. At first glance the left heart border, although well defined at the left atrial appendage (open black arrow), becomes indistinct suggesting adjacent lingula pathology. In the absence of previous imaging, a limited CT was performed (inset image) which confirms the appearance is due to a prominent fat pad (open white arrow).

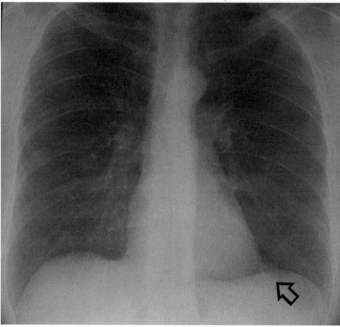

Figure 4.45. Cardiophrenic angle.

There is a 3 cm lesion in the region of the left cardiophrenic angle (open black arrow). Note the increased density has defined margins superiorly and medially that would not occur if due to a fat pad.

4.4 Pitfalls

4.4.1 Pseudo-pneumothorax

Any line that follows the contour of the chest wall may give the impression of a lung edge, implying the presence of a pneumothorax. Two instances to be aware of are the linear pleural thickening resulting from a previous chest drain (see *Fig. 4.46*), and AP mobile CXRs (see *Fig. 4.47*) which are taken with the patient lying against the X-ray plate to hold it in position. In the case of the AP film, the skin of the back may fold generating an air / soft tissue interface that subsequently appears on the CXR and mimics the lung edge seen in a pneumothorax (*Fig. 4.46*). Unlike a true pneumothorax, there will be lung markings visible beyond the apparent lung edge of a pseudo-pneumothorax.

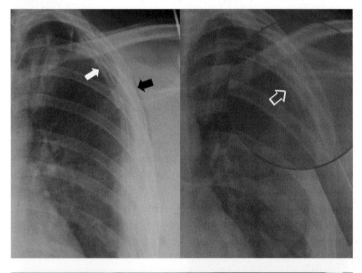

Figure 4.46. Pseudo-pneumothorax from chest drain.

Images from two CXRs combined. The right-hand image demonstrates a curvilinear line mimicking a lung edge (open white arrow). The cause is evident from the position of the *in situ* chest drain (white arrow) in the left-hand image. Note that there was a pneumothorax originally and the surgical emphysema can be seen on the left-hand image (black arrow).

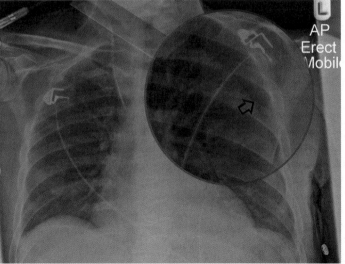

Figure 4.47. Pseudo-pneumothorax on a mobile AP film.

A mobile AP film demonstrating an apparent lung edge (open black arrow), but note that there are vessels beyond it. The edge is actually formed by a fold of skin on the patient's back as the patient is sitting semi-erect and the film cassette is against his back.

4.4.2 Patient rotation

The presence or absence of rotation is determined by comparing the projection of the spinous processes between the anterior ends of the clavicles. Rotation occurs around a central axis to which the clavicles are anterior and the spinous processes are posterior. Therefore, if the patient is rotated to the right the clavicle heads move to the right and the spinous processes to the left. On a properly centred CXR the spinous process will be projected equidistant between the anterior ends of the clavicles; rotation will result in the distance between the spinous process and the anterior ends of the clavicle being unequal, with the greater distance on the side to which the patient is rotated (*Fig. 4.48*).

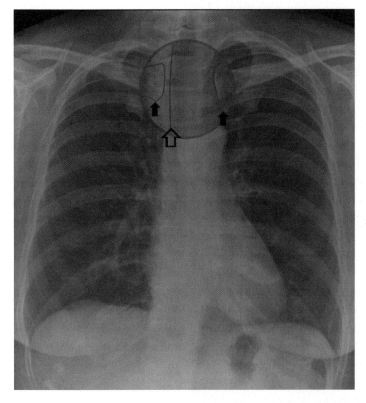

Figure 4.48. Rotation transradiancy.

The position of the spinous processes (open black arrows) compared to the medial ends of the clavicles (black arrows) reveals that this patient is rotated to the left. Note that there is a subtle increase in transradiancy of the left hemi-thorax, i.e. the side to which the patient is rotated.

The main reason for detecting rotation on a CXR is to explain apparent abnormalities that might otherwise be attributed to pathology. The transradiancy of the hemithorax to which the patient is rotated may be greater (i.e. the hemithorax appears darker) mimicking, for example, asymmetry in chest wall soft tissues, reduced vascularity, or increased density in the other hemithorax. The relative size and density of the hila may alter due to their different orientation, and apparent mediastinal shift toward the side to which the patient is rotated (the heart is an anterior structure in the chest) may mimic volume loss. Difference in rotation should always be considered when comparing two CXRs on the same patient (*Fig. 4.49*).

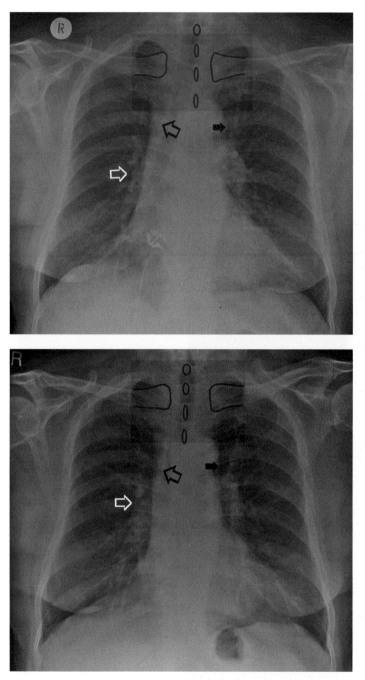

(a)

(b)

Figure 4.49. Rotation on CXR.

(a) Normal frontal CXR of an adult rotated to the right; note the relative positions of the spinous processes and ends of clavicles (outlined). Compare this with another CXR on the same adult (b), only this time rotated slightly to the left. Note the difference in appearance of the right hilum (open white arrow), paratracheal region (open black arrow), and descending aorta (black arrow).

4.4.3 Poor inspiration

There should be at least six anterior ribs visible superior to the hemi-diaphragms. More than six ribs may just indicate a good inspiratory effort rather than obstructive airways disease, which is better assessed in terms of flattening of the hemi-diaphragms (see later). If a poor inspiratory effort is made, the lower zones are most affected with crowding of the vessels causing increased density, physiological atelectasis, widening of the cardiac silhouette, and increase in apparent size and density of the hila. A poor inspiratory film should be interpreted with great caution (*Fig. 4.50*).

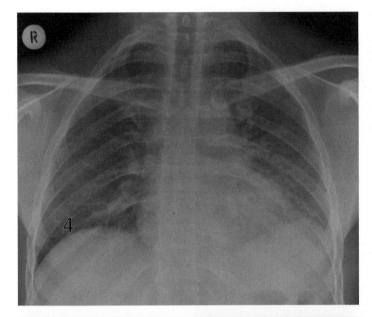

(a)

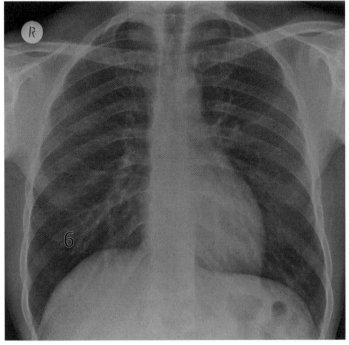

(b)

Figure 4.50. Effect of inspiratory effort.

Two normal frontal CXRs from the same patient; the numbers indicate the number of the lower-most anterior rib projected above the hemi-diaphragm. In image (a) there has been a sub-optimal inspiratory effort. As a result, the lungs appear more 'congested' and the hila more bulky when compared to image (b) where a good inspiratory effort has been made.

4.4.4 Mimics of nodules

Just as the silhouettes of the CXR are formed by aerated lung adjacent to soft tissue, any instance where soft tissue on the skin surface forms an interface with air, in line with the incident X-rays, will also form a silhouette. A dramatic example of this effect is the observation of multiple lesions on the skin of a patient with neurofibromatosis (*Fig. 4.51*).

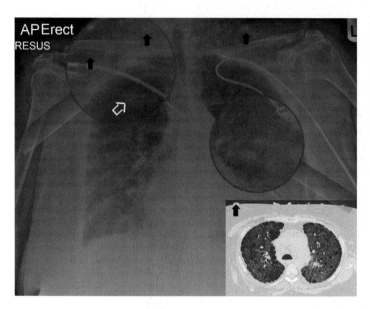

Figure 4.51. Neurofibromatosis.

AP CXR of a patient with neurofibromatosis; inset is an HRCT image. The lesions marked with black arrows are neurofibromas on the skin; where these overlay the lungs they mimic nodules in the lung (open white arrow). Note also the 'holes' in the lung on the CT image characteristic of neurofibromatosis involvement of the lung.

Similar in appearance, but far more common, are the apparent nodules simulated by the silhouette of the nipples. These can usually be identified by their position in relation to the breast contours, their symmetrical appearance, and a characteristic lack of definition to the supero-medial margin (*Fig. 4.52*).

If doubt remains, particularly if the appearances are asymmetrical, then a repeat film should be performed with the nipples marked by something radio-opaque. Similarly the use of nipple markers may confirm the appearances are not due to a nipple (see *Fig. 4.53*).

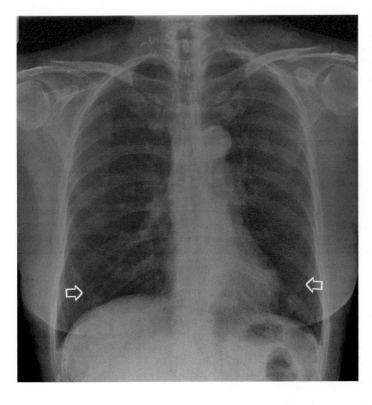

Figure 4.52. Nipple shadows.

Frontal CXR of an adult female. Both nipples are identifiable (open white arrow). Note the upper medial margin of the right nipple is not well defined.

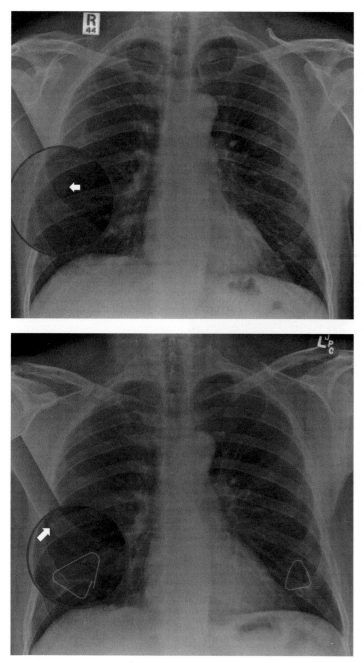

(a)

(b)

Figure 4.53. Nipple marking.

Frontal CXRs of an adult male. On the initial CXR (a) there is a possible soft tissue nodule felt most likely to represent a nipple shadow (white arrow) but a follow-up CXR with nipple markers (b) confirms that it is not a nipple. The degree of movement of the 'nodule' between the two CXRs despite only a minor amount of rotation indicates it is a surface abnormality and actually corresponded to a skin tag.

4.4.5 Pulmonary venous confluence

A minor anatomical variant of the draining of the pulmonary veins into the left atrium results in the joining of the superior and inferior pulmonary veins prior to entering the atrium. This pulmonary venous confluence (*Fig. 4.54*) can mimic a mass behind the right heart and may require further investigation; a limited CT scan usually resolves the issue.

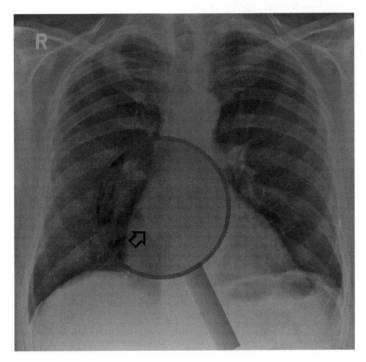

Figure 4.54. Pulmonary venous confluence.

Frontal CXR of an adult. Note the increased density behind the right heart in the magnified area (open black arrow). This corresponds to the pulmonary venous confluence where the pulmonary veins form a pseudo-chamber that then empties into the left atrium.

4.4.6 The manubrium sternae

The sternum overlies the mediastinum and has insufficient definition on a CXR to be discerned over the mediastinal density. However, the widest part of the sternum, the manubrium, corresponds to the narrowest, least dense part of the mediastinal silhouette and may therefore be seen overlying the trachea and adjacent structures. The lateral margins of the manubrium, when visible, may mimic para-tracheal lymphadenopathy, but careful scrutiny will reveal the characteristic shape of the manubrium.

The appearances when carefully observed will reflect a well-defined angular edge of appropriate shape (*Fig. 4.55*).

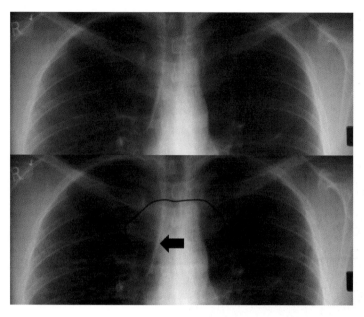

Figure 4.55. Manubrium.

In the top image there is increased density in the right superior mediastinum due to the manubrium. On the marked image the manubrium has been outlined; note the preservation of the right para-tracheal stripe (black arrow) indicating that there is no para-tracheal adenopathy to see.

4.4.7 Artefacts

Most surface artefacts can be identified for what they are without the need for further imaging. However, if doubt remains a repeat film with all possible artefactual objects removed should resolve the issue.

Clothing
A button or other potentially radio-opaque items on clothing can readily mimic soft tissue nodules. When solitary and overlying the lung the only indication that the appearances are artefactual may be the observation of regularly spaced holes for stitching the button into place (*Fig. 4.56*). When multiple, the artefactual nature is more readily appreciated with apparent nodules appearing in a line or even outside the confines of the lung (*Fig. 4.57*).

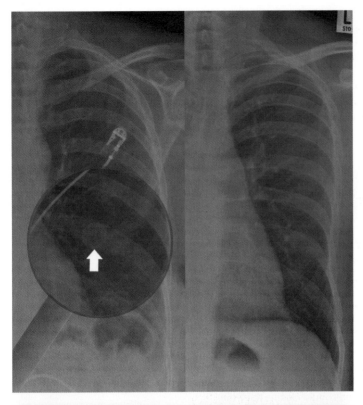

Figure 4.56. Button artefact.

The apparent nodule in the magnified area (white arrow) is a button. Careful scrutiny reveals the four stitching holes, but a follow up CXR (right image) was performed as a precaution and confirms the appearance was artefactual.

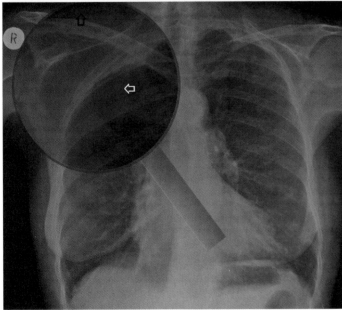

Figure 4.57. Clothing artefact.

Frontal CXR of an adult. There are multiple apparent nodules (open white arrow) but also multiple similar opacities (open black arrow) outside the chest. The abnormalities could potentially be skin-based, but in this case were due to sequins on a scarf.

ECG tabs

It is not unusual for ECG tabs to be left on patients when they are having a CXR (*Fig. 4.58*), and these artefacts can appear to be consistent over a series of films if they are left on the patient for any length of time. The CXR appearance is that of soft tissue density; the clue to their true nature is from the well-defined margins with rounded corners and their position with respect to the heart, especially if projected outside the chest. Again, repeat film with tabs removed should resolve the issue (see *Fig. 4.59*).

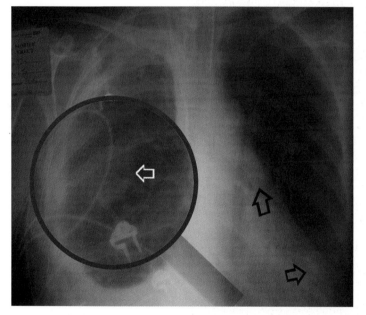

Figure 4.58. ECG tabs.

AP CXR of an adult. Note the numerous ECG tabs (open black arrows) and, in the magnified area, a further ECG tab that could easily be confused for a mass (open white arrow).

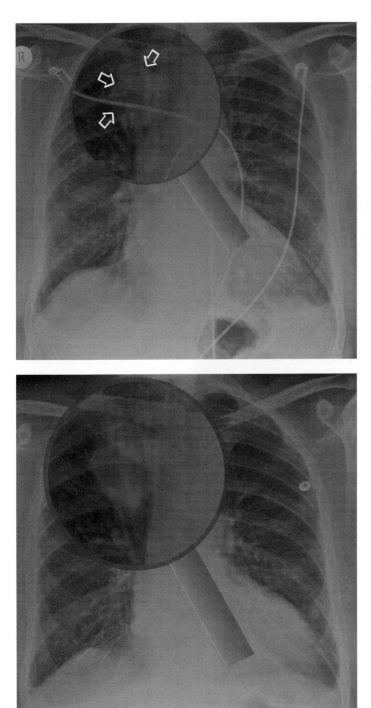

(a)

(b)

Figure 4.59. Opacity due to ECG tabs or cancer?

(a) Frontal CXR of an adult from cardiac pre-admission clinic. ECG leads are evident and it is not unreasonable to assign the opacity in the magnified area as being due to an ECG tab with what appear to be well defined, straight borders (open white arrows). The position of this supposed ECG tab was deemed to be a little high so a precautionary follow-up film with no surface artefacts was performed (b) and a primary lung cancer revealed.

Hair braids

Hair braids can cause disconcerting densities overlying the chest, particularly the apices (*Fig. 4.60*). As the braid originates from the head there will be no upper margin with the opacification extending above the chest; the stranding of the hair may trap air that is discernable on CXR. Repeating the CXR with the hair held out of the way will resolve the issue.

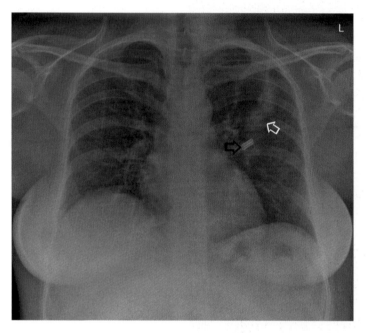

Figure 4.60. Hair braid on CXR.

The opacity projected over the left hemithorax is a hair braid (open white arrow). Note the hair band (open black arrow).

Film / screen and CR plate artefacts

Film screen (i.e. non-digital) systems use a material that fluoresces in response to incident X-rays and it is the resulting light that exposes the film. Foreign bodies such as dirt, dust and strands of hair, that are effectively transparent to X-rays when found on the fluorescing screen, will cast sharp shadows on the X-ray film as they are adjacent to the film being exposed by light, to which they are opaque (*Fig. 4.61*).

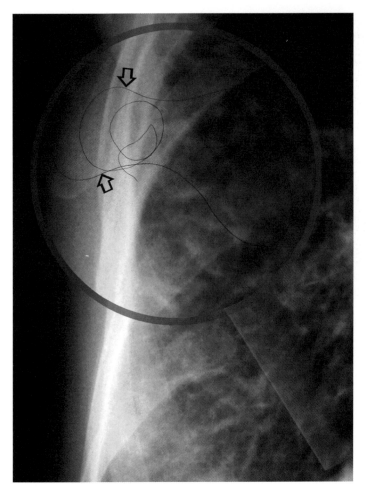

Figure 4.61. Hair on screen.

A magnified portion of a frontal CXR demonstrates the curvilinear opacity (open black arrows). Note that the contours are far sharper than other aspects of the CXR, such as the ribs. The cause is a hair trapped between the film and the screen.

CR film is only exposed to laser light after exposure to X-rays and removal from the cassette and is therefore less susceptible to artefacts due to foreign bodies on the film, but is susceptible to discrepancies due to film handling within the laser reader (*Fig. 4.62*). DR plates do not have a separate reading / digitising process and are therefore not susceptible to such artefacts.

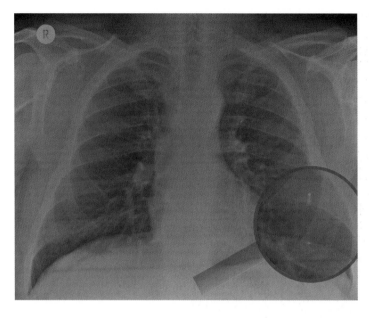

Figure 4.62. Roller artefact.

Frontal CXR of an adult taken using a CR digital system. Note the vertical linear artefact in the magnified area due to the handling of the digital plate in the reader.

05 Pattern recognition

The presence of apparent opacification in the lungs on a CXR will be due to one of the following: collapse, consolidation, ground glass opacification, nodules, reticulation/lines, lung mass, pleural mass/fluid/thickening, or increased chest wall tissue. By bearing these causes in mind and following the clues given below you should be able to interpret increased density, if not directly, then by a process of elimination.

5.1 Collapses

Collapse of a lobe or all of a lung is usually the result of obstruction to the relevant feeding airway. Due to the tapering nature of the bronchial tree, air may be able to escape from the lung but is prevented from entering it, and the remaining gases in the affected lobe are absorbed. Persistent aeration distal to a complete obstruction can occur as a result of collateral air drift, whereby air passes through links called 'pores of Cohn' found between adjacent secondary pulmonary lobules.

In the following descriptions the way in which the various lobes collapse is demonstrated, but note that the diagrams are for illustrative purposes to help describe the process of collapse; they do not in all instances represent the appearances one would see on a CXR. The key to understanding the collapses of the lobes is to understand the fissures separating the lobes and to remember that only air/soft tissue interfaces in line with the incident X-rays will generate a line on the CXR.

On the right there are two fissures: the oblique (major) fissure runs diagonally from posterior/superior to anterior/inferior, and the horizontal (minor) fissure runs horizontally and anteriorly from the point at which the major fissure crosses the hilum. The oblique fissure separates the right lower lobe from the right upper and middle lobes; any lung posterior to the oblique fissure is in the lower lobe. The horizontal fissure separates the right upper lobe superiorly from the right middle lobe inferiorly.

On the left there is no horizontal fissure. The bronchi to the lingula, which is the left-sided equivalent of what on the right is called the middle lobe, arise from the left upper lobe bronchus and therefore behave as part of the left upper lobe. The left oblique fissure takes a similar course to the right oblique fissure and is fixed at the hilum.

5.1.1 Right upper lobe collapse

The right upper lobe (RUL) collapses medially and anteriorly (*Figs 5.1–5.3*).

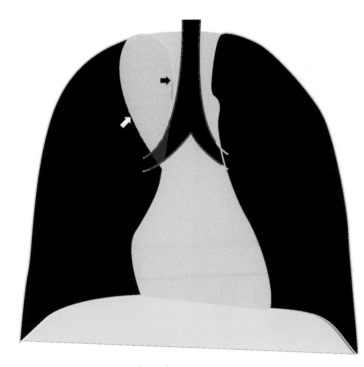

Figure 5.1. Right upper lobe collapse.

(a) On the PA view, the white arrow marks the minor fissure separating the right upper lobe from the over-expanded right middle lobe, and the black arrow highlights the loss of distinction between the collapsed upper lobe and the mediastinum as they are now of similar density.

(b) The lateral view shows that the loss of volume due to the collapse of the right upper lobe is mainly accommodated by an over-expansion of the right lower lobe, causing the upper lobe to collapse anteriorly, which causes the supra-hilar portion of the oblique fissure (white arrows) to move forward. There is also elevation of the minor fissure (black arrow) but, as is evident from the PA view, the movement of the minor fissure is primarily medial.

(a)

(b)

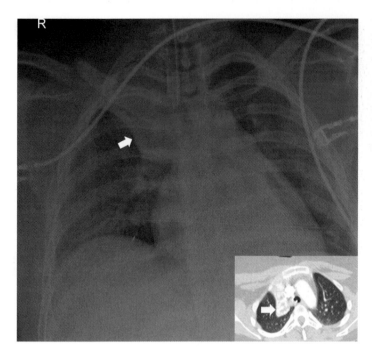

Figure 5.2. AP CXR of an ITU patient.

Mucous plugging has caused right upper lobe collapse. Note the elevation of the minor fissure (white arrow, also marked in the inset axial CT image), and the elevated right hemi-diaphragm due to the loss of volume. The lobe collapses anteriorly and has therefore obscured the para-tracheal stripe. Alternatively, the right lower lobe may over-expand to compensate and result in a spreading out of the right lower lobe vessels.

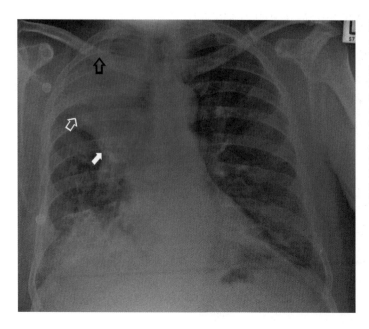

Figure 5.3. Right upper lobe collapse due to a central obstructing tumour mass.

The minor fissure is raised (open white arrow) indicating some collapse of the right upper lobe. There is increased opacity in the right apex and volume loss evident, with deviation of the trachea to the right; the cause for the collapse is the mass at the right hilum (white arrow). The combination of partial collapse and a central obstructing mass creates a curve to the minor fissure termed the 'Golden S sign'. Note the aerated lung in the apex (open black arrow) where the lower lobe is over-expanded to accommodate the collapsed upper lobe.

5.1.2 Left upper lobe collapse

The left upper lobe (LUL) collapses anteriorly like the right upper lobe. However, the lingula, the anatomical equivalent of a left middle lobe, is also involved *(Fig. 5.4)*. There is no minor fissure to elevate and move medially to demarcate the collapse, so this movement is added to that already necessary from the major fissure. Therefore, both the supra- and infra-hilar portions of the major fissure move forward and medially. As a result the lateral margin of the collapsed LUL fails to become orientated, such that a line is visible on the PA CXR *(Fig. 5.5)*, a role taken by the minor fissure in the case of a RUL collapse. The increased density of the collapsed LUL manifests as a veil-like opacification in the upper half of the left hemithorax; it becomes less dense towards the apex where the increasing proportion of aerated over-expanded LLL replaces the collapsed LUL, resulting in normal density at the apex and returns the overall density on CXR to normal. As the lingula is no longer aerated, the left cardiac silhouette is obscured. See *Figure 5.6* to see the effects of right upper and middle lobe collapse for comparison with LUL collapse.

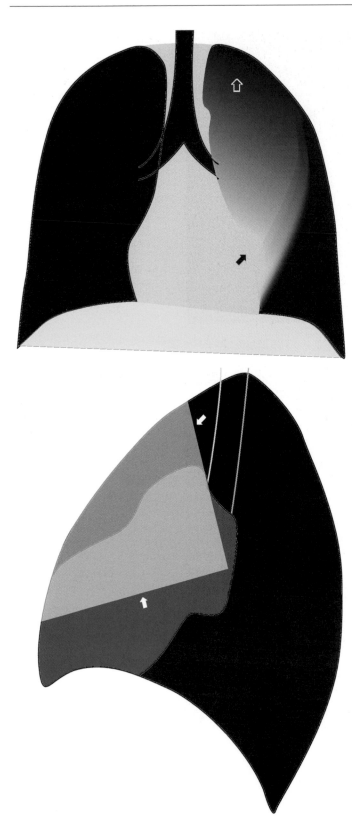

(a)

(b)

Figure 5.4. Diagrams of LUL collapse.

(a) Diagrammatic representation of a LUL collapse including the lingula. The inclusion of the lingula results in the increased opacification extending down to the left heart border, which is obscured (black arrow). There is no minor fissure so there is no clearly defined lateral margin (white arrow). Over-expansion of the lower lobe leads to almost normal density in the left apex (open black arrow). (b) The lateral view shows the demarcation on the collapsed LUL by the major fissure (white arrows), effectively tethered at the hilum.

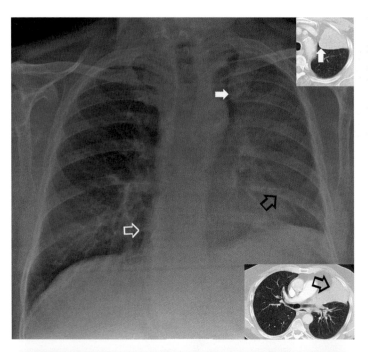

Figure 5.5. Frontal CXR of an adult with left upper lobe collapse.

Two axial CT images are inset. Note the opacification in the left hemithorax, obscuring the left heart border (open black arrow), the mediastinal shift to the left (open white arrow), and the margin between the over-expanded lower lobe and the collapsed upper lobe seen on the CXR and demonstrated on the inset CT image in the top right-hand corner (white arrow).

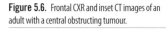

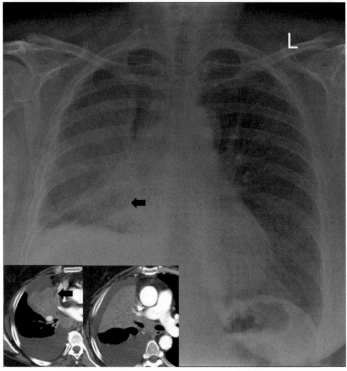

Figure 5.6. Frontal CXR and inset CT images of an adult with a central obstructing tumour.

The tumour has caused right upper and middle lobe collapse, which together are effectively the right-sided anatomical equivalent of the LUL (including the lingula). Note the loss of the right heart border (black arrow).

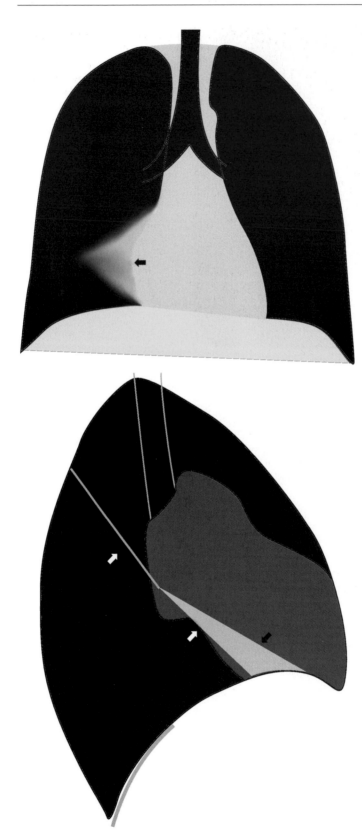

(a)

(b)

Figure 5.7. Diagrams of RML collapse.

(a) Diagrammatic representation of an RML collapse. The minor fissure is no longer orientated in line with the incident X-rays: it has moved downwards and medially and is therefore no longer visible on the frontal view. The right heart border is obscured by collapsed lung (black arrow).

(b) In the lateral view, movement of the minor fissure accommodates most of the loss of volume (black arrow) with compensatory expansion of the upper lobe and little movement of the major fissure (white arrows).

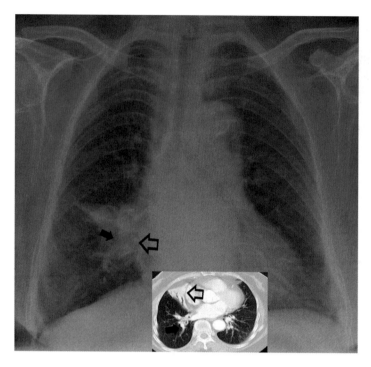

Figure 5.8. Frontal CXR and inset axial CT image of an adult with RML collapse.

Note the loss of clarity of the right heart border (open black arrow) and the visibility of the basal pulmonary artery (black arrow) through the opacity.

5.1.3 Right middle lobe collapse

The right middle lobe (RML) collapses inferiorly and medially (see *Fig. 5.7*), primarily accommodated by movement of the minor fissure which, in doing so, is no longer in the correct orientation to be seen on a PA CXR. As the RML is no longer aerated and lies adjacent to the heart, the right cardiac silhouette is obscured (*Fig. 5.8*).

5.1.4 Right lower lobe collapse

The right lower lobe (RLL) is bordered by the chest wall and the major fissure; it collapses inferiorly and medially, tethered at the hilum but pulling the hilum down and medially (*Fig. 5.9*). The supra-hilar part of the major fissure is pulled down, the infra-hilar part is pulled posteriorly, and both parts are pulled medially such that the orientation of the fissure at some point is in line with the incident X-rays of a PA CXR and is therefore discernable. The result is increased density in the right lower medial area of the right hemithorax, partially behind the heart and demarcated laterally by a border formed by the re-orientated major fissure. Over-expansion of the RUL and RML accommodates the space and the right hemi-diaphragmatic silhouette is usually preserved as the over-expanded RML comes to lie adjacent to the relevant part of the hemi-diaphragm (*Fig. 5.10*).

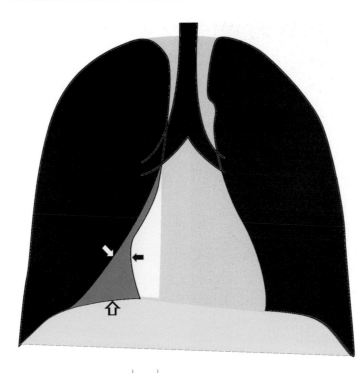

(a)

(b)

Figure 5.9. Diagrams of RLL collapse.

(a) Diagrammatic representation of the frontal view of an RLL collapse. The major fissure is drawn medially and now forms a silhouette (white arrow); the lobe collapses posteriorly such that the right heart border is unaffected (black arrow) and, if complete, the collapsed lower lobe lies sufficiently posterior to allow the RML to preserve the right hemi-diaphragmatic silhouette (open black arrow). (b) The lateral view demonstrates the movement of the major fissure (white arrows) and minor fissure (black arrow) effectively tethered at the hilum; note the aerated expanded RML now lies adjacent to the right hemi-diaphragm, thus preserving the silhouette.

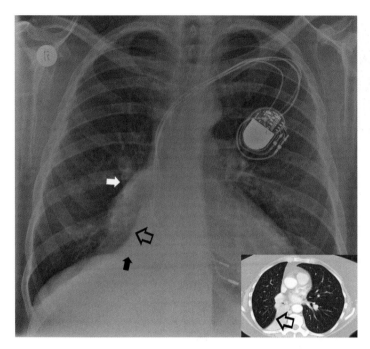

Figure 5.10. Frontal CXR and inset axial CT image of an adult with a three chamber cardiac pacemaker and a right lower lobe collapse.

Note the silhouette formed by the collapsed lobe (open black arrows). The hilar point is depressed (white arrow) and the right hemi-diaphragmatic silhouette is preserved (black arrow). Comparison of the lower zones will reveal a relative reduction in vascularity at the right base as the lung here is over-expanded, spreading out the vascular markings.

5.1.5 Left lower lobe collapse

Collapse of the left lower lobe (LLL) occurs in the same way as that of the RLL (see *Fig. 5.11*). The main differences are that the increased density lies entirely behind the heart, making it more difficult to perceive, and the medial aspect of the left hemi-diaphragmatic silhouette is usually lost in LLL collapse (*Fig. 5.12*); the apex of the left hemi-diaphragm that generates the diaphragmatic silhouette lies more posteriorly on the left compared to the right, because of the heart, and is therefore more likely to be obscured by a collapsed LLL.

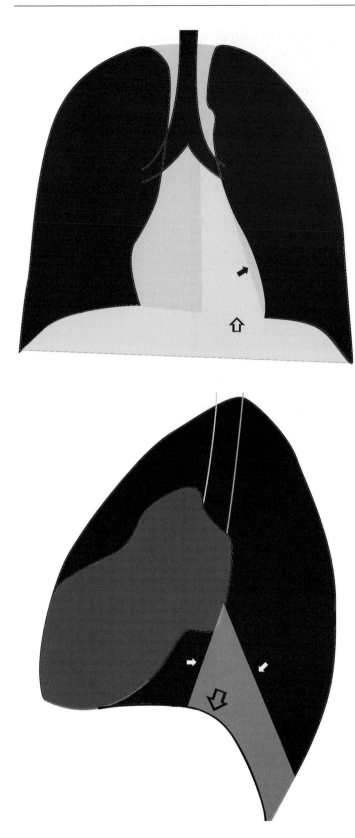

Figure 5.11. Diagrams of LLL collapse.

(a) Diagrammatic representation of an LLL collapse. Note that, as for the RLL collapse, the oblique fissure is pulled into line with the incident X-rays demarcating the lateral margin of the collapsed lobe. The medial left hemi-diaphragmatic silhouette is obscured more readily than in the case of an RLL collapse, because the presence of the heart causes the uppermost margin of the hemi-diaphragm that gives rise to the silhouette to arise more posteriorly (open black arrows).

(b) As for the RLL collapse, the lateral view shows that the oblique fissure is tethered at the hilum, effectively bending but also, as is evident on the frontal view, folding medially. The more posterior diaphragmatic apex is involved during the collapse.

(a)

(b)

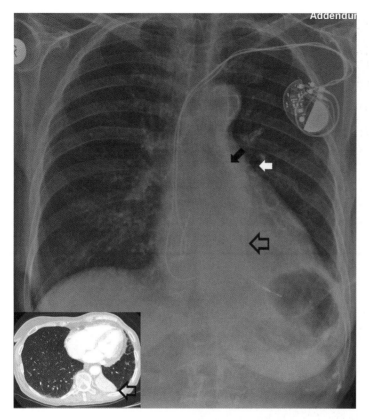

Figure 5.12. Frontal CXR and axial CT inset of an adult with a cardiac pacemaker and LLL collapse.

Note the depression of the left main bronchus (black arrow) and the hilar point (white arrow), loss of the medial hemi-diaphragmatic silhouette, and paucity of lung markings in the left mid / lower zone. The signs indicate lower zone volume loss with overexpansion of the remaining lung and identifies the lateral edge of the collapsed LLL (open black arrow) as the cause of the increased density behind the heart.

5.1.6 Whole lung and multiple lobe collapse

Collapse of an entire lung (*Fig. 5.13*) may occur quite suddenly secondary to an obstruction of the main bronchus. The lung volume decreases markedly and the mediastinal shift to the side of the collapse accommodates this loss of volume, but the degree to which the lung can collapse is limited by its attachment to the chest wall. In the case of a large pneumothorax the lung can collapse to the size of a large fist due to elastic recall, but the hemithorax cannot accommodate collapse to that degree. Without air-flow the air in the lung is replaced by fluid causing diffuse opacification of the hemithorax. This replacement by fluid is surprisingly rapid and presumably the result of negative intra-thoracic pressure on inspiration, drawing fluid into the lung in the absence of any in-flow of air.

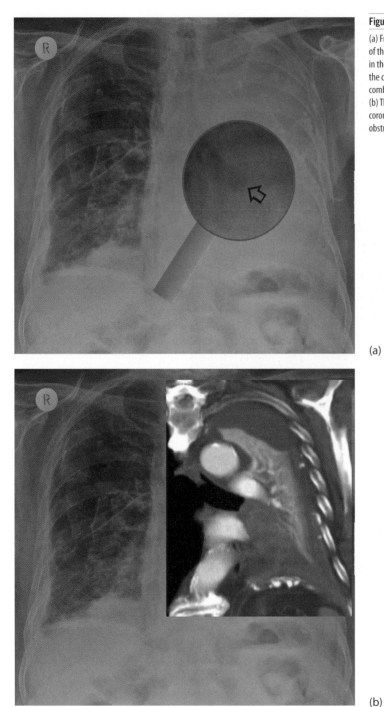

Figure 5.13. Collapse of the left lung.

(a) Frontal CXR of a patient with complete collapse of the left lung, secondary to an obstructing tumour in the left main bronchus (open black arrow). Note the complete opacification of the left hemithorax combined with mediastinal shift to the left.
(b) The same CXR with part of a CT-generated coronal reconstruction overlaid to demonstrate the obstructing tumour.

(a)

(b)

5.2 Ground glass opacity

Initial filling of the air spaces, displacing the air, results in an increase in density of the lung, such that there is insufficient density difference between the vessels and the partially aerated lung to be distinguished on CXR; the vessels are therefore obscured and this is termed ground glass opacity (see *Fig. 5.14*). Note that the contrast resolution of CT is far greater than CXR and the same process on CT imaging gives an increased density without obscuring the vessels.

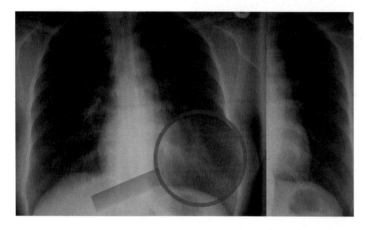

Figure 5.14. Ground glass opacity.

The magnified area highlights ground glass opacity in the lingula obscuring the left heart border. For comparison, the right-hand image taken 6 weeks after antibiotic therapy demonstrates resolution of what was pneumonia.

5.3 Consolidation

Consolidation describes the complete filling of the air spaces in the lung with radio-dense material; in simplistic terms the 'material' concerned is pus (pneumonia), blood (haemorrhage, or aspiration), water (left heart failure, acute lung injury, etc.), or cells (cancer). The small airways are the last to fill as material accumulates in the alveolar air spaces first (*Fig. 5.15*); normally these airways are not visible as their walls are too thin to show up on CXR and they contain, and are surrounded by, air. When the surrounding lung is consolidated, the contrast between the air in the airway and the now opacified lung makes these smaller airways visible as black lines (air-bronchograms, see *Figs 5.16* and *5.17*). As consolidated lung is no longer aerated any adjacent silhouette is lost, not only highlighting the consolidation but also localizing it (*Figs 5.18* and *5.19*). However, the silhouette is only affected if the consolidation is in the area of lung that contributes to a silhouette (*Fig. 5.20*).

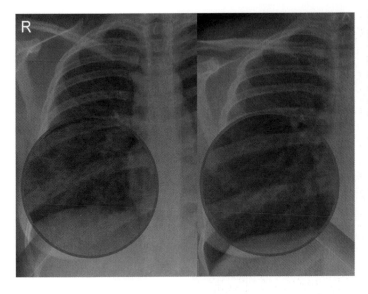

Figure 5.15. Portions of two frontal CXRs on the same adult presenting with symptoms of infection.

The image on the left shows increased opacification with a nodular appearance; an earlier normal CXR is shown on the right for comparison. This is developing consolidation, but the opacification of the lung has yet to become uniform and create air-bronchograms.

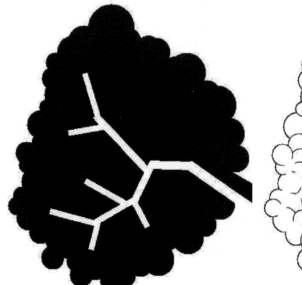

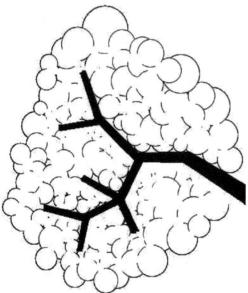

Figure 5.16. Consolidation of a lung.

The left hand image is a diagrammatic representation of a pulmonary lobule. The vessels (white) are seen contrasted with the aerated lung (black); the accompanying small airways are not visible. When the lung is no longer aerated, right hand image, the vessels are obscured; the contrast is now between the air in the small airways (black) and the opacified lung (white); this is consolidation.

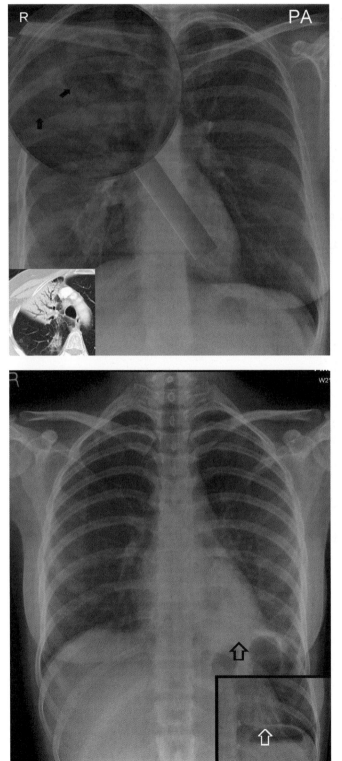

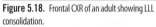

Figure 5.17. Frontal CXR showing consolidation with part of a CT image inserted.

There is consolidation in the RUL; note the air-bronchograms (black arrows) and the same appearance on the CT image.

Figure 5.18. Frontal CXR of an adult showing LLL consolidation.

The inset image is from a CXR taken 3 weeks earlier. Note the loss of the medial left hemi-diaphragmatic silhouette (open white arrow) due to segmental LLL consolidation (open black arrow).

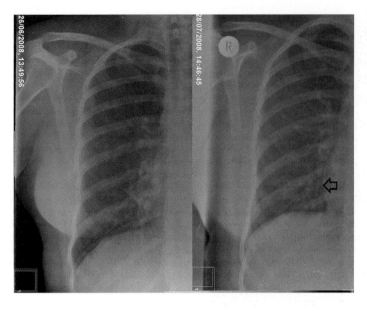

Figure 5.19. Sections from two frontal CXRs of the same adult taken 4 weeks apart showing RML consolidation.

Note the loss of clarity of the right heart border due to consolidation in the RML.

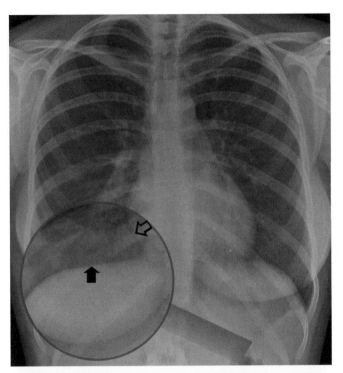

Figure 5.20. Frontal and lateral CXRs of an adult with RLL consolidation.

(a) In the magnified area of the frontal CXR there is an area of opacification obscuring the vessels, but with preservation of the diaphragmatic (black arrow) and right heart border (open black arrow) silhouettes.
(b) The lateral view explains the appearances: the apex of the right hemi-diaphragm (black arrow) giving rise to the silhouette clearly lies anterior to the portion of hemi-diaphragm adjacent to the consolidation (open white arrow).

(a)

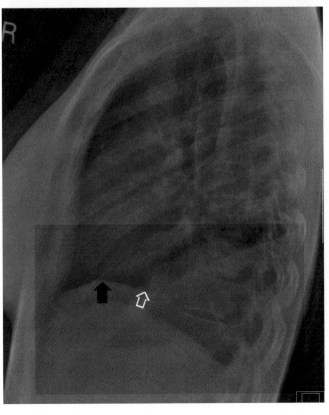

(b)

5.4 Masses

An opacity measuring 3 cm or more in diameter is termed a mass. Clues to the pathology of a mass may be gleaned from its density, margins, position and rate of growth.

5.4.1 Density

High density areas seen on CXR would indicate calcification. In masses, calcification is a less reliable indicator of a benign pathology than in smaller nodules because matrix calcification in larger cancers is not uncommon. However, the nature of the calcification may be of diagnostic value: 'popcorn' calcification (large clumps of calcification forming in cartilage) is found in hamartomas, but note that cartilage containing sarcoma metastases may also have popcorn-like calcification. Low density masses are rare and difficult to interpret with confidence on CXR; the presence of a significant amount of fat is a good indicator of underlying benign disease.

5.4.2 Margins

The margins of a mass on CXR depend upon the integrity of the adjacent aerated lung. If the mass is purely displacing lung tissue one would expect it to have well-defined margins; if the pathology is infiltrating, or replacing aerated lung, or surrounded by ground glass opacity, or consolidation, then the relevant margins are likely to be less well defined (*Fig. 5.21*).

The loss of the margin of a mass due to an adjacent soft tissue structure will indicate where in the chest that mass is located. The presence of a well-defined medial margin and no lateral margin suggests a pleurally based location and is a result of the curved nature of the chest (*Fig. 5.22*). Pleurally based masses sited anteriorly or posteriorly in the chest may have no defined margins in the correct orientation to be seen on a CXR and are only apparent as a subtle change in density. If there is evidence of chest wall involvement then the location of a mass is readily determined (*Fig. 5.23*). A mass arising from or abutting the mediastinum will not have a well-defined medial margin and is likely to alter the mediastinal silhouette (*Figs 5.24 and 5.25*).

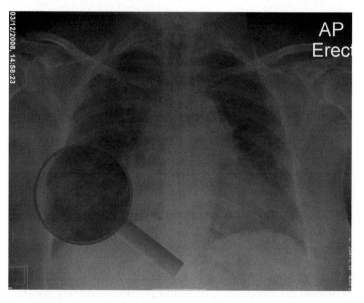

Figure 5.21. Frontal CXR of an adult patient with a primary lung cancer.

At presentation the tumour is indistinct with ill-defined margins.

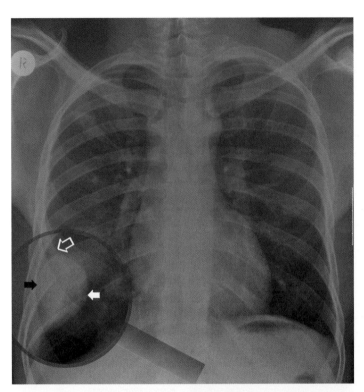

Figure 5.22. Frontal CXR showing a pleurally based mass.

Note the absence of a defined lateral margin (black arrow), a well-defined medial margin (white arrow) and an obtuse angle with the chest wall (open white arrow).

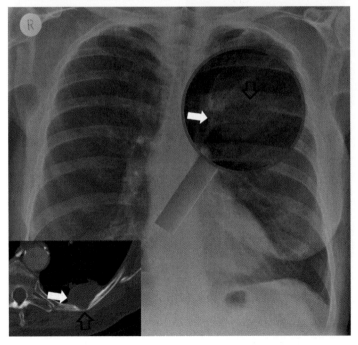

Figure 5.23. Pleural lesion to rib.

In the magnified area is a soft tissue mass (white arrow). Only the inferior margin is well seen. Note the associated erosion of the underlying rib identifying this lesion as being posteriorly based and highly likely to be malignant. These features are also highlighted on the CT image insert.

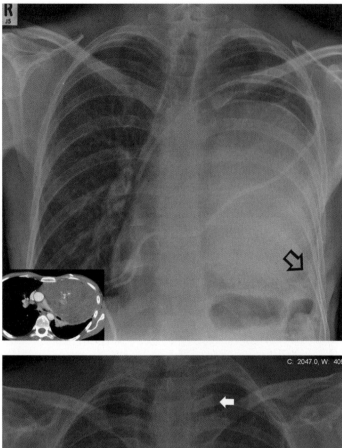

Figure 5.24. Frontal CXR of an adult with a large anterior mediastinal mass (see inset image).

Note there is no left mediastinal contour to see and the mass in this case is so large that the left hilum has been displaced posteriorly and cannot be seen on the CXR. Note that there is lower density in the region of the costophrenic angle (open black arrow) where there is some aerated left lower lobe contributing to the overall density.

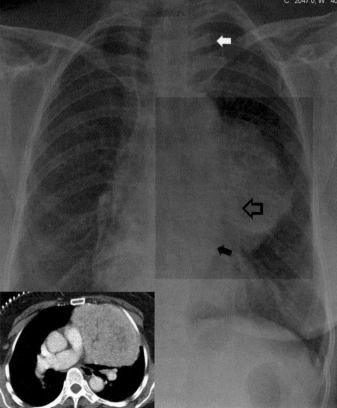

Figure 5.25. Frontal CXR and inset axial CT of an adult with a large thymoma.

Note the mass obscures the left heart border (open black arrow) but the silhouettes of the hila and descending aorta (black arrow) are preserved. In addition there is superior extension of the tumour into the thoracic inlet mimicking a goitre (white arrow).

Masses may hide behind the diaphragm in the posterior costophrenic recess, in the apices and in the para-spinal region projected behind the heart (see *Section 4.3.5*).

5.5 Nodules

Nodules measure less than 3 cm in maximum diameter and may be solitary or multiple (see *Table 5.1*); the likely cause may be determined by considering their size, density, distribution and multiplicity, and considering the patient's clinical status.

Table 5.1. Causes of multiple nodules

Size	Density	Distribution	Disease
<5 mm	Soft tissue	Widespread	Miliary TB
			Fungal infection
		(more in bases)	Hypersensitivity pneumonitis
		Mid zones	Coal miner's pneumoconiosis
		Mid zones	Sarcoid
		Basal	Fibrosing alveolitis
	High density	Widespread	Haemosiderosis
			Siderosis
			Stannosis
			Alveolar microlithiasis
		Mid zones	Silicosis
			Barytosis
2–5 mm	Soft tissue	Widespread and discrete	Carcinomatosis
			Lymphoma
			Sarcoidosis
		Widespread and tend to confluence	Pneumonia (e.g. TB)
			Pulmonary oedema
		Basal and tend to confluence	Hypersensitivity pneumonitis
		Peripheral and tend to confluence	Fat emboli

Size	Features	Distribution	Disease
>5 mm	Calcification, cavitation dependent on cell type	Widespread	Metastases
	Cavitation common	Widespread	Abscesses
	Cavitation and calcification	Upper lobes	Coccidiomycosis
	Few in number, may calcify	Any	Histoplasmosis
	Cavitation, well defined	Widespread	Wegener's
	Cavitation	Lower zones, peripheral	Rheumatoid nodules
	Cavitation, calcification, background pneumoconiosis	Any	Caplan's syndrome
	Well defined, lobulated	Any	Arterio–venous malformation

Vessels viewed end on will mimic the appearance of nodules and determining whether there really are nodules in the lung can prove difficult. Clues can be gleaned from the size of the apparent nodules: the vessels are of smaller calibre the more peripheral they are; if the apparent nodules are consistently of the same diameter as the nearby vessels, then they are likely to represent vessels end on. In the extreme periphery of the lung the vessels are too small to be seen on CXR; therefore nodules in these regions are real. The best area to scrutinise for the periphery of the lung is the space between the projections of the anterior and posterior ribs (*Fig. 5.26*). See *Figures 5.27–5.32* for examples of CXRs showing a range of nodule types.

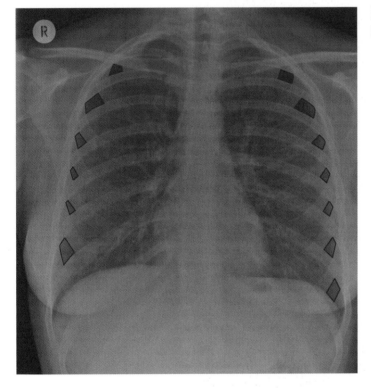

Figure 5.26. Normal frontal CXR highlighting the peripheral regions where the ribs do not overlap.

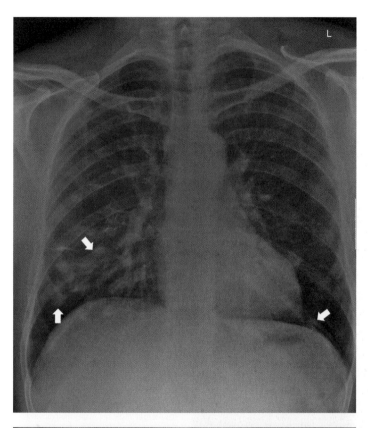

Figure 5.27. Frontal CXR demonstrating multiple soft tissue nodules of varying size.

The main diagnosis to exclude is that of metastases. In this case the patient was undergoing chemotherapy for leukaemia and the nodules were shown on biopsy to represent histoplasmosis, a fungal infection.

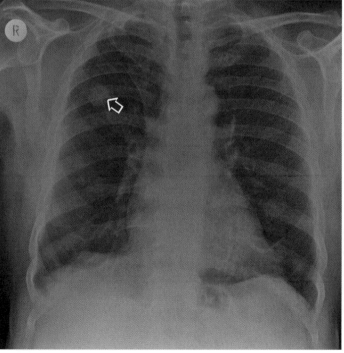

Figure 5.28. Frontal CXR on an adult smoker with a solitary pulmonary nodule.

The nodule can be seen in the right upper zone (open white arrow). Note also the azygos fissure. This nodule was resected and found to be an adeno-carcinoma.

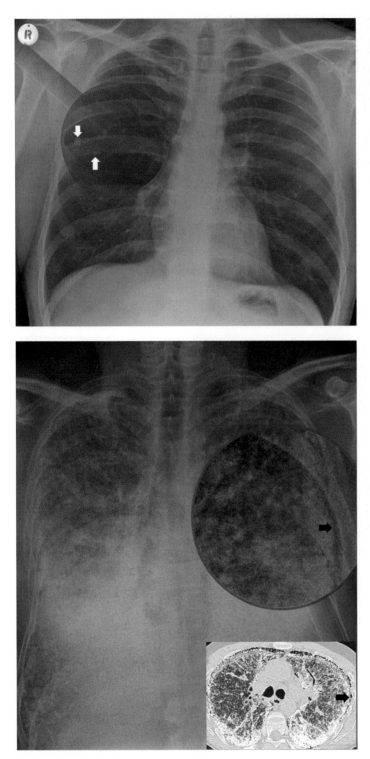

Figure 5.29. Frontal CXR of a patient with previous pulmonary chickenpox.

The numerous variable sized granulomata are calcified and are therefore easy to identify despite being small.

Figure 5.30. Frontal CXR of an adult with a markedly abnormal CXR but clinically asymptomatic.

In the magnified area you should be able to see that the cause for the diffuse increase in density is multiple very small nodules; for nodules of this size to be visible on CXR they must comprise a dense material, in this case small stones of calcium within the alveoli. Note the black pleura sign (black arrow) where the lung has no stones. The CT image (inset) demonstrates the diffuse nature of the abnormality, but the stones themselves are too small to be seen on CT.

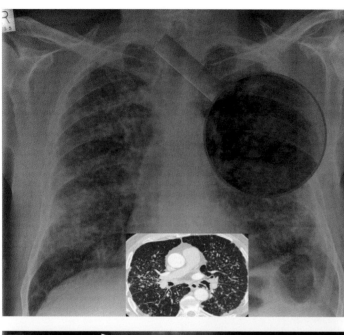

Figure 5.31. Frontal CXR and inset axial CT image of an adult with silicosis.

Note the extensive nodularity.

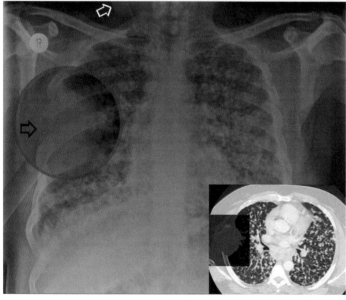

Figure 5.32. Frontal CXR and inset axial CT of an adult with metastatic thyroid cancer.

This could easily be a case of TB as there is diffuse miliary nodularity, soft tissue opacification associated with destruction of the right fourth rib (open black arrow), and cervical lymphadenopathy (open white arrow).

5.6 Lines

There are four basic types of lines on the CXR and these are described in this section.

5.6.1 Band shadowing / atelectasis

Band shadowing (*Fig. 5.33*) is most commonly seen towards the lung bases. Parenchymal bands result from atelectasis (collapse) of a sub-segmental portion of lung usually found following focal pneumonia, pulmonary embolism or general anaesthetic. Note that the terms band shadow and atelectasis are usually interchangeable; band shadowing is the term that tends to be used when the line on the CXR is thicker.

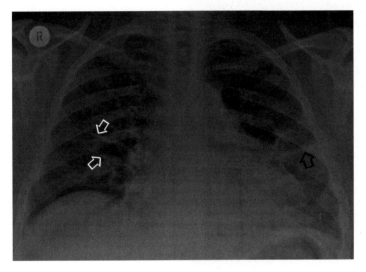

Figure 5.33. AP CXR on a post-operative patient.

There is band shadowing (open black arrow) and atelectasis (open white arrows).

5.6.2 Curvilinear

Curvilinear lines are found in bullous emphysema (*Fig. 5.34*). The entire margin of the bulla is rarely if ever seen but parts of the wall may cross the X-ray beam at the correct angle to create a line on the CXR.

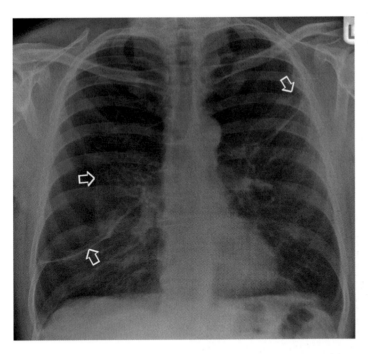

Figure 5.34. Frontal CXR of an adult with bullous emphysema most marked in the right upper lobe.

Note the paucity of vessels in the right upper and mid zones and the curvilinear lines (open white arrows) corresponding to the walls of bullae. Note also that the entire bullous wall is not usually discernable.

5.6.3 Septal lines (Kerley A, B lines)

Septal lines (*Fig. 5.35*) are caused by the accumulation of fluid or other material in the interlobular septa. Kerley B lines are found at the periphery of the lung bases; they are 1–2 cm in length and extend at right angles from the pleural surface. The commonest causes are left heart failure and lymphangitis carcinomatosa, but septal lines may also be seen in pneumoconiosis and sarcoid. Kerley A lines are the result of the same process as Kerley B lines, but are seen radiating out from the hila.

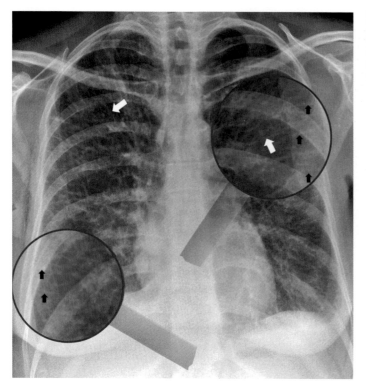

Figure 5.35. Frontal CXR in a patient with heart failure.

Note the Kerley B lines (black arrows) readily seen up to the mid zones and the longer Kerley A lines radiating from the hila (white arrows).

5.6.4 Reticulation

Reticulation represents thickening of the lung interstitium and is difficult to identify with confidence on a CXR. The pattern consists of criss-crossing fine lines, which must be distinguished from the normal vascular pattern. Potential causes are fluid accumulation in the interstitium, such as in pulmonary oedema, or thickening due to cellular or fibrotic processes. As the interstitium extending to the surface of the lung is usually the first to become affected, reticulation is often better appreciated at the periphery of the lung on the CXR, and the now visible interstitium of the lung adjacent to soft tissue structures interferes with the silhouette sign, resulting in an irregular or ill-defined margin (*Fig. 5.36*).

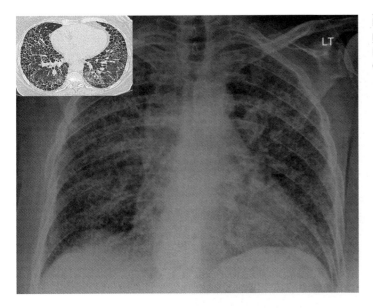

Figure 5.36. Frontal CXR of an adult with idiopathic pulmonary fibrosis.

Note the reticulation causing obscuration of the diaphragmatic and mediastinal silhouettes.

5.7 Cavities

A cavity is the development of an air space within solid tissue, whether a mass (*Fig. 5.37*), nodule, consolidation or infarcted lung (*Fig. 5.38*); because the cavity lies within an area of abnormal tissue it will have a thicker wall than found in cysts or bullae. As inflammatory cavities heal they may become thinner walled and more cyst-like (see *Section 8.1* on pulmonary TB).

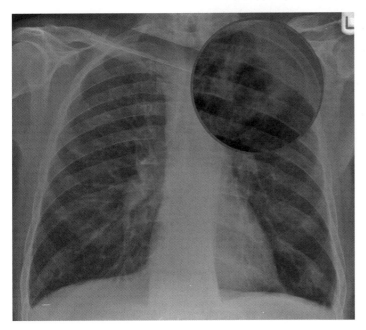

Figure 5.37. Frontal CXR of a patient with squamous cell carcinoma.

Note in the magnified area a soft tissue mass with central cavitation. Of the primary lung cancers, squamous cell carcinoma is the most likely to cavitate.

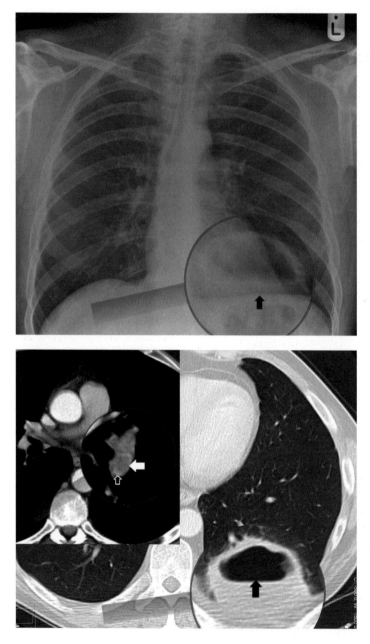

(a)

(b)

Figure 5.38. Cavitating infarct.

(a) Frontal CXR of an adult with a large cavitating lesion in the left lower lobe; note the preservation of the hemi-diaphragmatic silhouette (black arrow). (b) CT image of the same cavity containing a fluid level (black arrow) and an inset demonstrating contrast in the left basal pulmonary artery (open white arrow) surrounding an embolus (white arrow). Although the cavity is secondary to infarction resulting from a large pulmonary embolus, the presence of a fluid level suggests additional infection.

06 Abnormalities of the thoracic cage and chest wall

6.1 Pectus excavatum

Pectus excavatum (*Fig. 6.1*) occurs as an isolated phenomenon but is also strongly associated with Marfan's syndrome. The physical abnormality is a depression of the sternum and anterior chest wall; this causes an alteration in the orientation of the ribs which are more horizontal posteriorly and more vertical anteriorly, and which is classically described as a number 7 shape. The heart is pushed to the left such that the right heart border overlies the spine and is poorly defined. Pectus may be surgically corrected but the procedure has limited success.

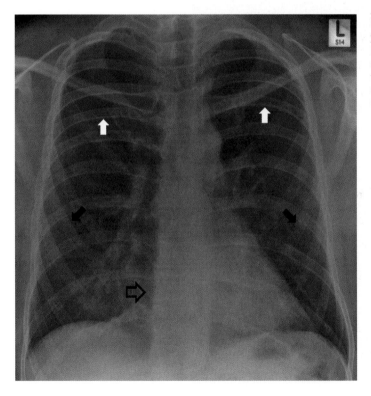

Figure 6.1. Frontal CXR of a young male with pectus excavatum.

Note the abnormally steep angle of the anterior ribs (black arrows), the horizontal orientation of the posterior ribs (white arrows) and the indistinct right heart border with mediastinal shift to the left (open black arrow).

6.2 Scoliosis

Scoliosis is curvature of the spine in the coronal plane; it should be straight at rest. The thoracic spine can normally flex laterally such that a scoliosis on CXR may be due to poor patient positioning; a natural response to unilateral musculoskeletal chest pain is to 'splint' the area of pain, contracting the local muscles and causing lateral flexion of the spine. In such cases the degree of curvature is minor, but in congenital conditions scoliosis can be dramatic (*Figs 6.2* and *6.3*).

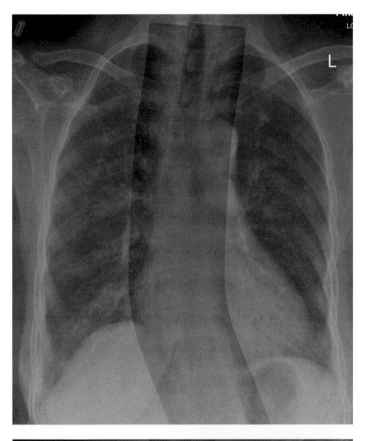

Figure 6.2. Frontal CXR of a patient with a thoracic scoliosis concave on the left.

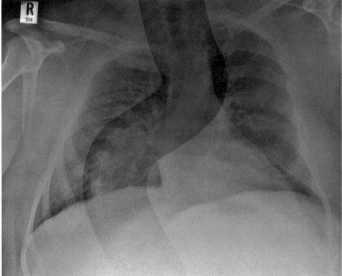

Figure 6.3. AP CXR of an adult patient with a dramatic biconcave congenital scoliosis.

The curvature of the spine is highlighted in the contrast-enhanced region.

Scoliosis may also indicate intrinsic spinal pathology such as degenerative disc disease, facet joint sclerosis or asymmetric loss of vertebral height.

The thoracic spine should be visible on a CXR and careful scrutiny of the para-spinal lines may indicate whether there is an acute spinal pathology, such as a fractured vertebra with adjacent haematoma, or osteomyelitis with an adjacent abscess.

6.3 Kyphosis

The spine in the sagittal plane is not straight but forms a double S shape. Mechanically this enables the spine to absorb impacts along its length, e.g. whilst running, by minor degrees of flexion and extension at each intervertebral joint. The thoracic spine has a physiological kyphosis.

An accentuation of the thoracic kyphosis may have an impact on respiratory function by restricting chest expansion. This is difficult to appreciate on a frontal CXR, although clues exist such as the chin overlying the upper mediastinum, the lower projection of the clavicles, and the more vertical orientation of the ribs. A lateral CXR is the best way to appreciate the extent of any accentuated kyphosis and to identify the commonest cause, which is a wedge collapse of one or more vertebral bodies (*Fig. 6.4*).

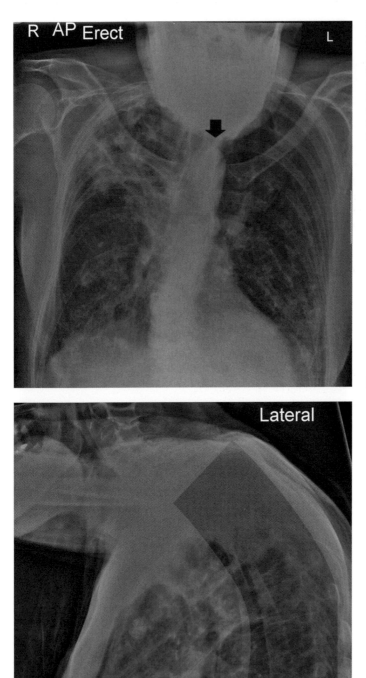

Figure 6.4. Kyphosis shown on AP and lateral CXR.

(a) AP CXR of an adult with marked kyphosis. Note the vertical orientation of the ribs and the projection of the chin over the superior mediastinum.

(b) Lateral view of the same subject with the curvature of the spine highlighted; the cause was mid-thoracic wedge collapses secondary to osteoporosis.

(a)

(b)

6.4 Bone lesions

In general, primary tumours of the bone are far less common than metastatic deposits from primary tumours elsewhere and this is true of the thoracic cage. In addition, there are non-malignant pathologies that may produce focal or diffuse bony abnormalities.

The superimposition of the lung vasculature over the anterior and posterior ribs makes interpretation of rib abnormalities difficult; the vessel markings mimic lucencies and, in the absence of cortical erosion or endosteal scalloping, lucencies should be diagnosed with caution. The identification of sclerotic lesions is more straightforward (*Fig. 6.5*) but still prone to errors in interpretation. In addition, a diffusely sclerotic skeleton may be overlooked when there is no normal bone for comparison (*Figs 6.6* and *6.7*). Lesions in the ribs are best appreciated in the lateral ribs where there is no superimposed lung; lesions here can be diagnosed with far greater confidence. It is worth noting that the ribs are often overlooked when a CXR is viewed as, in order to view the lungs, one learns to ignore the ribs; turning the CXR 90° alters the orientation of the ribs such that they no longer conform to the pattern normally seen on a CXR and may be scrutinised and appreciated more easily (*Fig. 6.8*).

It is important to remember that the clavicles scapulae, proximal humeri and the spine are all imaged on a CXR, and lesions in these sites, perhaps with the exception of the spine, are easier to interpret than those in the ribs but are often overlooked (see Figs *6.9, 6.10* and *6.11*). Non-malignant lesions of the bones may be evident on a CXR and may provide clues as to the cause of a patient's symptomatology. Findings as simple as rib fractures, new or healing, may explain pleuritic chest pain.

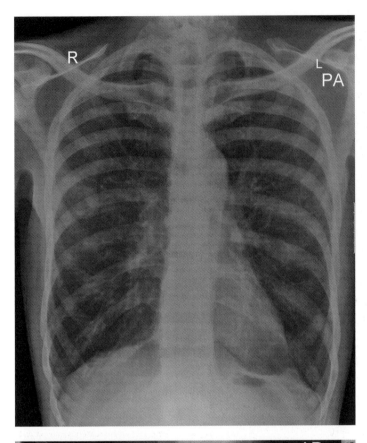

Figure 6.5. Frontal CXR of a male patient with sclerotic prostatic metastases.

There are no magnified areas because it is a general overview of the chest that demonstrates the widespread areas of increased bone density.

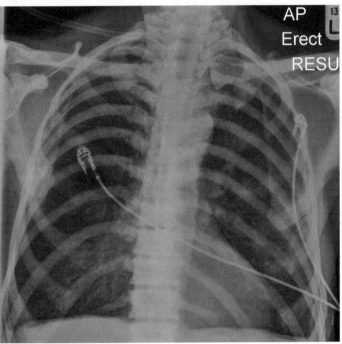
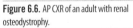

Figure 6.6. AP CXR of an adult with renal osteodystrophy.

The skeleton is diffusely sclerotic; note the loss of differentiation between the cortex and the endosteal region of the ribs.

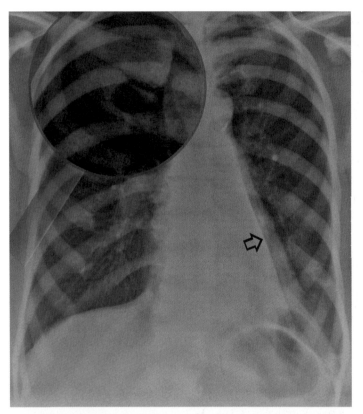

Figure 6.7. Frontal CXR of an adult female.

Note again the diffuse increase in density of the bones and, more evident in this example, loss of the normal cortical medullary differentiation (magnified area). There are some lucencies too and the edge of a collapsed LLL can be seen (open black arrow). The cause of the sclerosis in this case is from a rare manifestation of multiple myeloma, the LLL collapse resolved spontaneously.

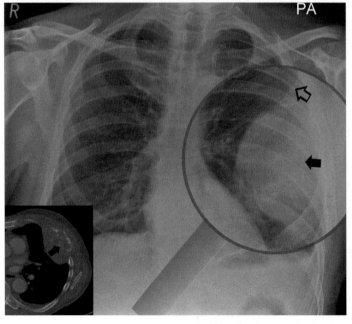
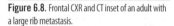

Figure 6.8. Frontal CXR and CT inset of an adult with a large rib metastasis.

Note the destruction of the anterior left rib (black arrow); the obtuse angle (open black arrow) made by this mass with the lateral chest wall favours a chest wall or pleural origin for this lesion.

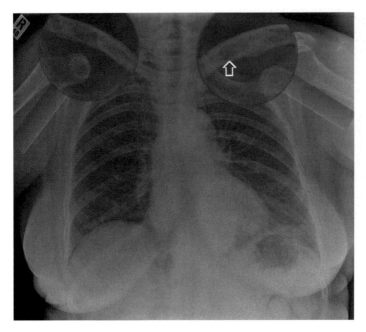

Figure 6.9. AP CXR of an adult female with multiple myeloma.

Note the lucencies in the clavicles with endosteal scalloping (open white arrow); numerous other lucencies can be seen following careful scrutiny.

Non-malignant lesions of the bones may be evident on a CXR and may provide clues to the cause of a patient's symptomatology. Findings as simple as rib fractures, new or healing, may explain pleuritic chest pain (*Figs 6.10* and *6.11*).

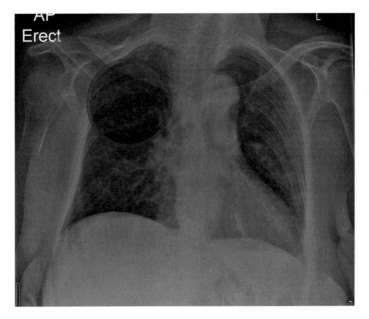

Figure 6.10. Frontal CXR of an adult with renal cell carcinoma.

In the magnified area there are numerous nodules of varying size which are also apparent elsewhere in the lungs, but did you notice the abnormality of the humerus due to a destructive bony metastasis?

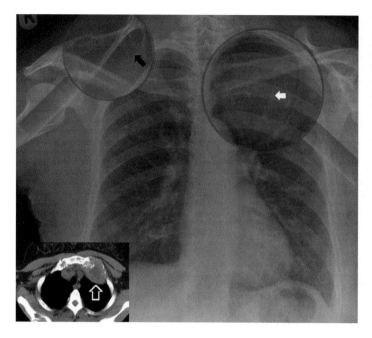

Figure 6.11. Frontal CXR and axial CT inset of an adult with metastatic cancer.

Increased opacity in the left apex, not obscuring the vessels (white arrow), is due to a large rib metastasis (open white arrow). In addition there is a further metastasis in the right scapula (black arrow).

6.5 Chest wall / thoracic inlet

Prominent lesions on the skin surface may be of sufficient density to be seen on CXR, particularly if they are surrounded by air giving them a well-defined margin. The true nature of these lesions may be apparent from their projection outside the confines of the lung and / or identifying the lesions themselves on the patient's body. The neurofibromas found in neurofibromatosis are a dramatic example of such 'nodules' (*Fig. 6.12*). Soft tissue masses in the chest wall may be apparent through asymmetry in the contours of the soft tissue of the chest (*Figs 6.13* and *6.14*). If the increase in chest wall soft tissue lies anterior or posterior to the lungs, it causes a difference in density without obscuring the underlying intra-thoracic structures. Note bilateral symmetrical chest wall masses may be perceived in the presence of breast prostheses which are not always immediately apparent (*Fig. 6.15*).

The soft tissue structures of the chest wall should be roughly symmetrical; the transradiancy (overall darkness / lightness) of the hemithoraces should be compared and any difference needs to be explained. The commonest cause for a difference in transradiancy is rotation of the patient, in which case the difference is artefactual and the increased transradiancy is seen on the side to which the patient is rotated. Any asymmetry in the soft tissues of the chest wall can cause a discrepancy in transradiancy, e.g. Poland's syndrome (congenital absence of pectoralis muscle), hemiplegia or polio causing muscle wasting, and mastectomy causing an increase in transradiancy (*Fig. 6.16*), and soft tissue thickening due to tumour or inflammation causing a decrease in transradiancy (see *Fig 6.14*).

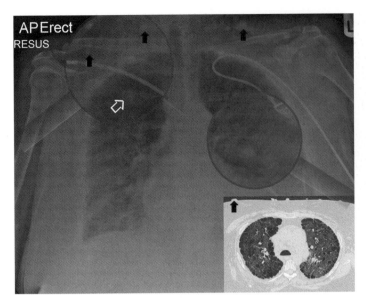

Figure 6.12. Frontal CXR with axial CT image inset of an adult with neurofibromatosis.

Note the numerous cutaneous neurofibromas (black arrows) easily identified on the skin surface. More difficult to interpret are the neurofibromas overlying the lungs (open white arrow) appearing to be soft tissue nodules. The already indistinct margins are projected over the interstitial oedema, paraseptal emphysema, and additional parenchymal air-filled cysts (these are described in neurofibromatosis) in the underlying lung (see inset image).

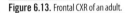

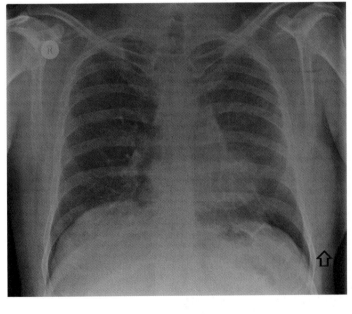

Figure 6.13. Frontal CXR of an adult.

Note the difference in the contours of the lateral chest wall. The mass (black arrow) was a haematoma at a recent thoracoscopy site.

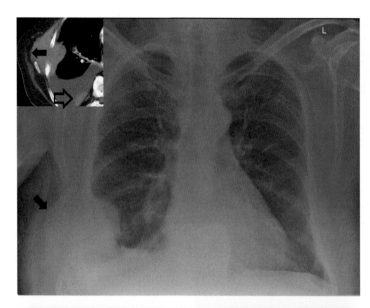

Figure 6.14. Frontal CXR and inset CT image of an adult with pleural adenocarcinoma metastases (open black arrow).

One of the pleural metastases has eroded into the chest wall and its lateral margin can be seen (black arrow).

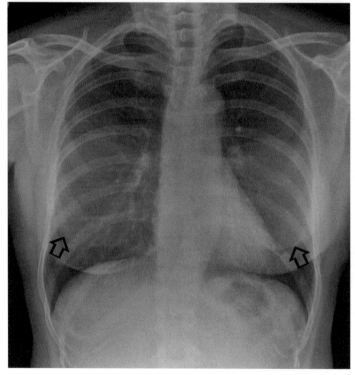

Figure 6.15. Frontal CXR of an adult female with bilateral breast implants.

The breast implants (open black arrow) cause increased density but with no effect on the underlying silhouettes.

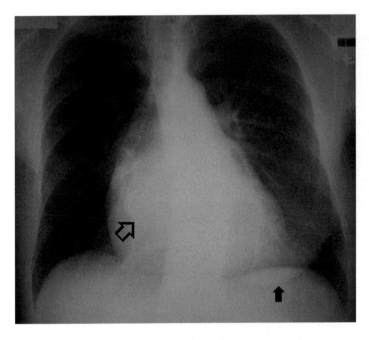

Figure 6.16. Frontal CXR of an adult with a right mastectomy and mitral valve disease.

Note the intact left breast shadow (black arrow) and the enlarged left atrium (open black arrow).

6.6 Thoracoplasty

An historical treatment for pulmonary TB was the surgical collapse of the affected lobe depriving what is an aerobic organism of oxygen. Although a reasonably effective treatment at the time these patients suffered from respiratory failure in later life (*Fig. 6.17*).

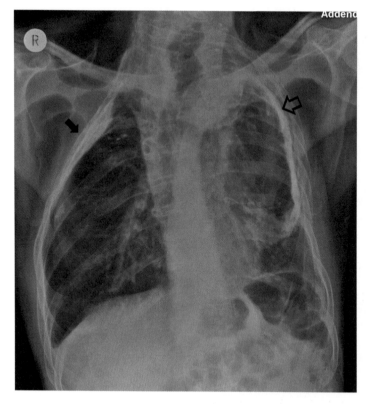

Figure 6.17. Frontal CXR of an adult treated in the past for pulmonary TB with a thoracoplasty.

The marked deformity of the thoracic cage (black arrow) is iatrogenic in origin; the dense pleural calcification (open black arrow) is due to previous TB empyema.

07 Lung tumours

7.1 CXR features of malignant tumours

7.1.1 Ill-defined / spiculated margins

The assumption that poorly defined margins or spiculation equates to an invasive pathology is based upon the premise that infiltration of the adjacent lung causes a loss of clarity in the margins of the lesion, indicating malignant invasive disease (*Fig. 7.1*). To some extent this is true, but inflammatory processes can be ill-defined for the same reason and malignant tumours that primarily metastasise via lymphatics and blood vessels may not have local invasion as a major component and subsequently have well-defined margins.

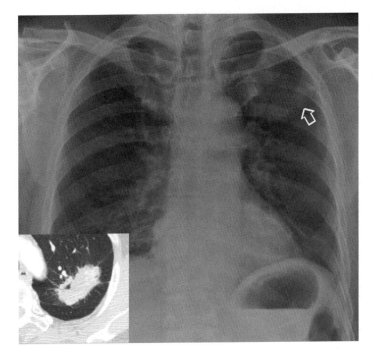

Figure 7.1. Frontal CXR and inset CT image of an adult with lung cancer in the left upper lobe.

Note on the CT image the spiculated margin to this lesion; as a result, despite its size, the margins are ill-defined (open white arrow).

7.1.2 Rapid increase in size

Tumour growth rates are best measured in terms of the time taken to double in volume. It is important to realise that a doubling in volume will only result in a 24% increase in diameter and that it is difficult to exclude malignancy on the grounds of a too rapid increase in size, although most lung tumours have a volume-doubling time of between 4 and 13 months (*Figs 7.2* and *7.3*).

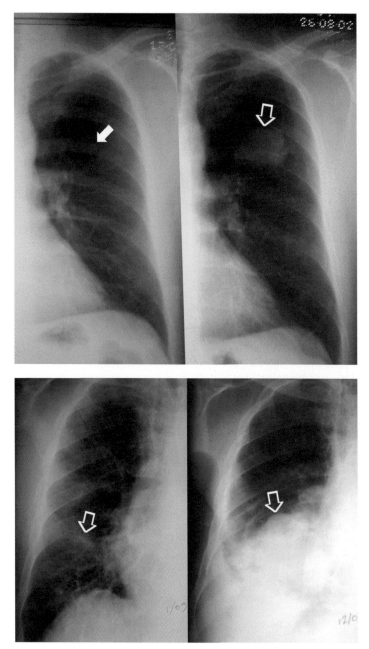

Figure 7.2. Selected portions of two CXRs taken 30 months apart.

The mass (open white arrow) has grown from the nodule (white arrow).

Figure 7.3. A portion of two CXRs of the same adult taken 11 months apart.

The primary lung cancer missed on the initial CXR as it is obscured by underlying pulmonary fibrosis has grown rapidly (open white arrow).

7.1.3 Erosion of adjacent rib

Erosion of an adjacent rib confirms the peripheral position of the mass and invariably indicates malignancy (*Fig. 7.4*); osteomyelitis resulting in an inflammatory mass or abscess could mimic this but is less likely.

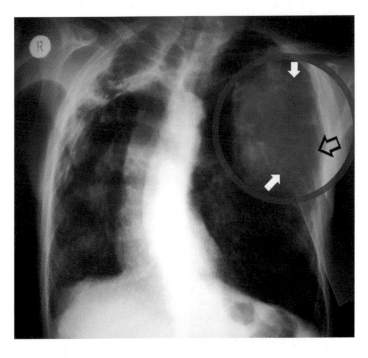

Figure 7.4. Frontal CXR of an adult demonstrates opacification in the left upper zone.

Note that the malignant nature of this lesion is evident from the destruction of the adjacent rib (open black arrow); the other adjacent ribs (white arrows) are as yet not involved.

7.1.4 Presence of hilar / mediastinal adenopathy

Hilar and/or mediastinal adenopathy increase the suspicion of malignancy in the context of a lung mass / nodule (*Fig. 7.5*), but there are numerous benign causes for such a combination, particularly tuberculosis and sarcoid (*Fig. 7.6*).

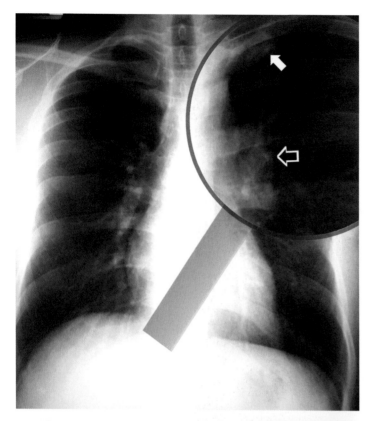

Figure 7.5. Frontal CXR of an adult with primary lung cancer and hilar adenopathy.

In the magnified area the primary lesion is difficult to discern hidden behind the first costo–chondral junction (white arrow). The hilar adenopathy (open white arrow) is more obvious and in this case increases the index of suspicion for there being a primary lesion in the left lung.

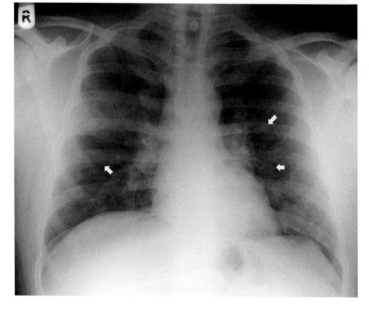

Figure 7.6. Frontal CXR of an adult with multiple nodules of variable size (white arrows) and bilateral hilar adenopathy.

Despite the malignant feel to this CXR, the cause for the appearances is sarcoidosis.

7.1.5 Presence of a pleural effusion on the side of the lesion

In the context of a proven malignancy, the presence of a unilateral pleural effusion (*Fig. 7.7*) suggests pleural spread of disease, conferring a poor prognosis and removing the possibility of treatment with intent to cure. However, this is a poor predictor of malignancy in an undiagnosed lung lesion, because para-pneumonic effusions are common and the appearances may be entirely due to inflammation. Even in the presence of a known malignancy the pleural fluid should be sampled to confirm malignant involvement before potentially curative management is discarded.

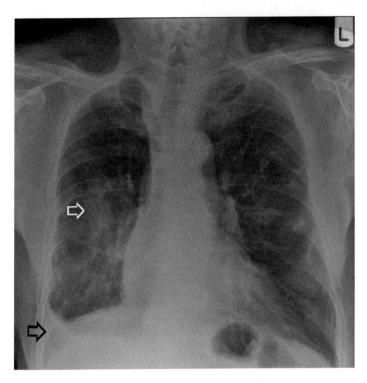

Figure 7.7. Frontal CXR on an adult with an adenocarcinoma of the lung (open white arrow).

Associated with this is a unilateral pleural effusion (open black arrow), which is suspicious for a malignant effusion. In this case the effusion was confirmed to contain malignant cells, making the tumour irresectable.

7.1.6 Evidence of lymphangitis carcinomatosa

Tumour infiltration of the lymphatic system in the lungs causes interstitial thickening and congestion resulting in reticulation and septal lines. In the context of a mass lesion, the appearance of lymphangitis carcinomatosa would indicate underlying malignancy (*Fig. 7.8*), but similar appearances may be due to a bulky benign tumour obstructing the proximal lymphatic system, or increased pressure in the lymphatics due to heart failure. A marked unilateral lymphatic congestion is less likely to be the result of heart failure.

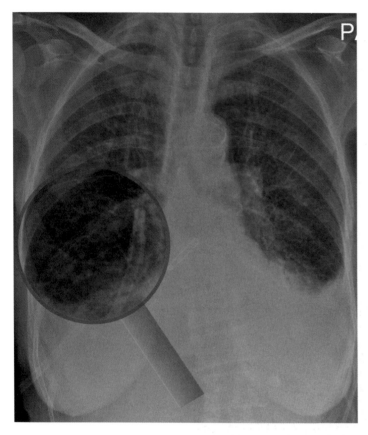

Figure 7.8. Frontal CXR of an adult patient with disseminated adenocarcinoma and lymphangitis carcinomatosa.

Note the numerous septal lines and the bilateral pleural effusions, both of which contained malignant cells.

7.2 CXR features of benign tumours

7.2.1 Calcification

The commonest benign nodules in the lung are granulomata, usually from previous infection, particularly tuberculosis (*Fig. 7.9*). Another infective cause of calcified nodules is chickenpox pneumonia. Calcification identified in a nodule 2 cm or less is a reasonable predictor of benignity, particularly if the calcification is marked enough to be seen on CXR. Hamartomas are the commonest benign neoplasm in the lungs and they classically contain 'popcorn' type coarse calcification, but this can be difficult to appreciate on CXR (*Fig 7.10*). As always there is a cautionary note, because metastatic cartilage-forming tumours such as osteosarcoma may demonstrate matrix ossification (*Fig. 7.11*).

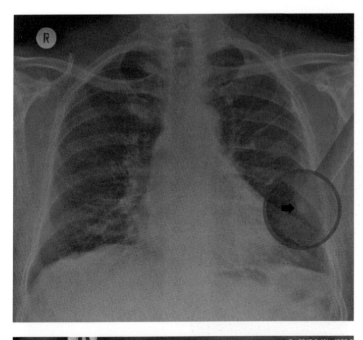

Figure 7.9. Frontal CXR of an adult who had TB as a child, resulting in a calcified granuloma in the lung (black arrow).

Soft tissue nodules of this size would be difficult to see on CXR, but when calcified they are, as in this case, clearly seen.

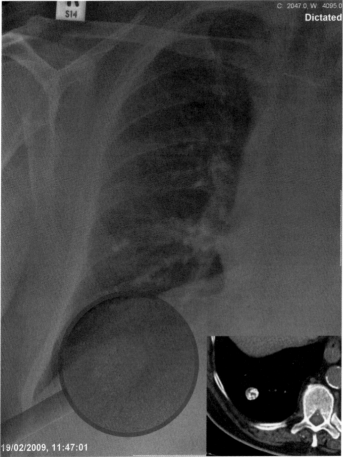

Figure 7.10. Part of a frontal CXR with an axial CT inset of an adult with a hamartoma.

The lesion is difficult to see behind the hemi-diaphragm, but has well-defined margins. The 'popcorn' calcification evident on the CT scan is not readily appreciated on the CXR.

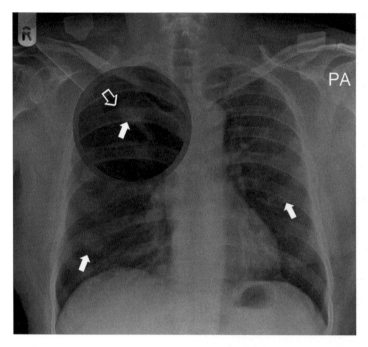

Figure 7.11. Frontal CXR of an adult male with osteosarcoma metastases (white arrows).

Note the density of these lesions, particularly the one in the magnified view, due to ossification. In addition there is a pneumothorax (open white arrow) which is a recognized complication of osteosarcoma metastases.

7.2.2 Low density, high fat content

Low density within a lesion, indicating a high fat content, is a strong predictor of benignity, typically a hamartoma (*Fig. 7.11*). The interface between fat and soft tissue is just discernable on a CXR, but in the context of a nodule the amount of fat is very unlikely to be sufficient to be detectable. A high fat content in a mass may be gleaned from the overall low density of the mass, but this would be a difficult judgement call; the greater contrast resolution of CT scanning will usually resolve such issues.

7.2.3 Slow or non-growing

Nodules identified on a CXR not demonstrating clear features of being benign are likely to undergo CT scanning and, if they do not contain fat or significant calcification, they will be followed up to ensure no growth over an 18 month to 2 year period. If a nodule identified on CXR is seen to be static in growth over at least a 2 year period, then a benign pathology is assumed; the availability of previous CXRs may demonstrate the static nature of the nodule and obviate the need for CT scanning and further follow up (*Fig. 7.12*).

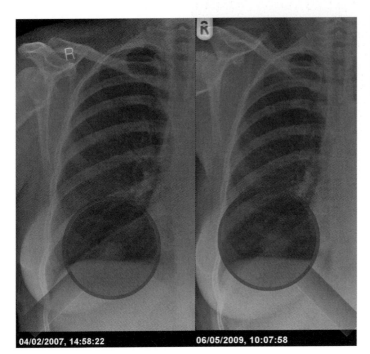

04/02/2007, 14:58:22   06/05/2009, 10:07:58

Figure 7.12. Sections from two frontal CXRs of an adult female presenting with an incidental finding of a nodule on CXR (magnified region).

Review of a previous CXR from over 2 years before indicates no growth and so no follow up is required. This is probably a hamartoma.

7.3 Metastases

Multiple soft tissue nodules of varying size are considered to be metastases until proven otherwise. Metastases tend to have well-defined margins, replacing rather than infiltrating the lung (*Fig. 7.13*), but some tissue types, adenocarcinoma in particular, can mimic focal consolidation creating ill-defined opacities.

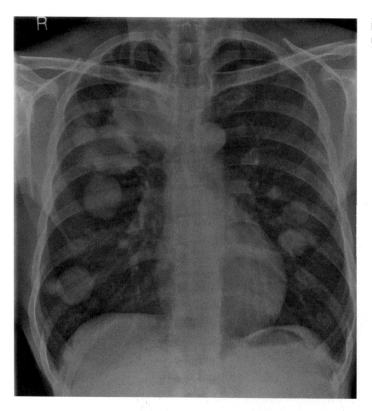

Figure 7.13. Frontal CXR of an adult with metastatic renal cell carcinoma.

Possible non-malignant causes for multiple nodules of varying size are sarcoidosis (*Fig. 7.6*), the vasculitides such as Wegener's granulomatosis, and some infections such as histoplasmosis (*Fig. 5.27*).

7.4 Bronchial carcinoma

For the purposes of treatment, bronchogenic carcinoma can be conveniently divided into small cell lung cancer (SCLC) and non-small cell lung cancer (NSCLC).

7.4.1 Non-small cell lung cancer

The tumours that comprise the NSCLCs are adenocarcinoma, squamous cell carcinoma and large cell carcinoma. These are difficult to distinguish with any degree of certainty on CXR, but cavitation strongly favours squamous cell carcinoma (*Fig. 5.37*), as does a more central location; adenocarcinomas are more commonly peripheral in position (*Fig. 7.14*) and may have a primarily consolidative appearance, as in alveolar cell carcinoma (*Fig. 7.15*). When located in the apex, a NSCLC is referred to as a pancoast tumour; these are easily overlooked and characteristically cause shoulder and arm symptoms due to invasion of the brachial plexus (*Fig. 7.16*).

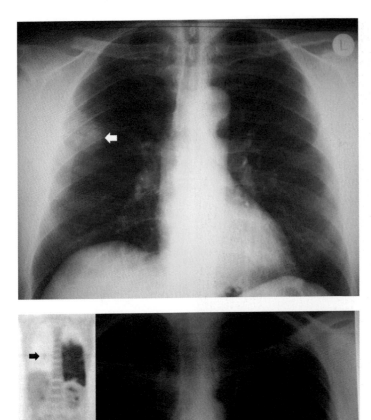

Figure 7.14. Frontal CXR of an adult with adenocarcinoma (white arrow).

This lesion was not visible on bronchoscopy and was diagnosed by percutaneous biopsy.

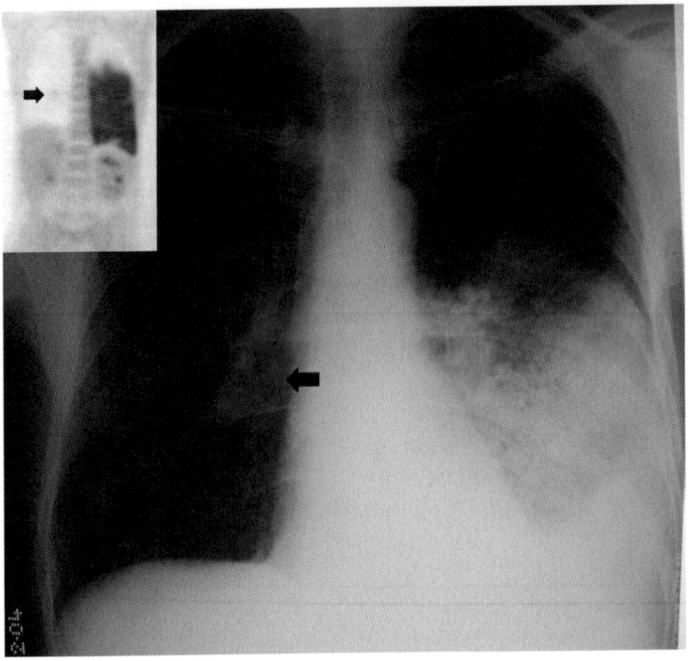

Figure 7.15. Frontal CXR of an adult with alveolar cell carcinoma occupying the majority of the left lower lobe.

The tumour is FDG avid and is therefore 'hot' on PET and a further smaller area in the contra-lateral lung (black arrow) indicates disease spread.

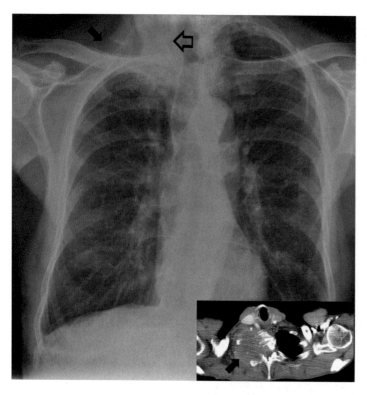

Figure 7.16. Frontal CXR and inset CT image of an adult with a pancoast tumour in the right apex.

Note the increased opacification (open black arrow) and the absence of the ribs through tumour erosion (black arrows).

7.4.2 Small cell lung cancer

SCLC behaves as a systemic disease and has usually spread extensively at presentation. The most characteristic presentation is with marked mediastinal lymphadenopathy; despite the large volume of metastatic disease, the primary tumour may be so small as to be overlooked. Surgical management of SCLC is not advocated and the prognosis is poor.

Distinguishing between NSCLC and SCLC on CXR is not possible but marked mediastinal lymphadenopathy, out of proportion to the size of the primary tumour, should increase suspicion for a SCLC (*Fig. 7.17*). Ultimately, as for all lung tumours, histology or cytological confirmation is required.

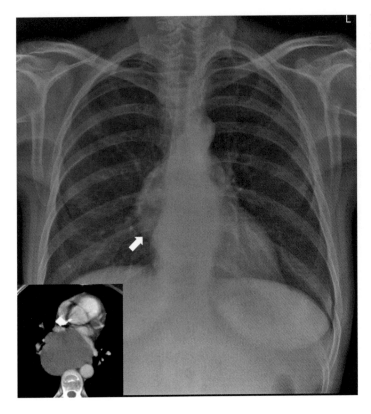

Figure 7.17. Frontal CXR on an adult patient with SCLC.

The unusual right mediastinal contour (white arrow) is due to massive sub-carinal adenopathy (inset).

7.5 The solitary pulmonary nodule

A solitary pulmonary nodule (SPN) identified on CXR can be managed in a systematic way.

1. Is it real? If there is any suspicion that the appearance may be due to overlapping shadows, surface artefacts or vessels end-on, then a repeat CXR possibly in a different orientation may resolve the issue. If a surface artefact is suspected (see *Section 4.4*) the CXR should be repeated ensuring only a gown is worn and that any cutaneous nodules are marked with a radio-opaque marker prior to the repeat CXR (to correlate the surface lesion with the CXR finding). If overlapping shadows (particularly ribs) or end-on vessels (nodule the same diameter as the adjacent vessels) are suspected, the orientation of the incident X-rays should be changed, such that the shadows are separated or the vessel orientation with respect to the incident x-rays is changed; the best way of achieving this is through a lordotic view (see *Section 4.3.1*).

2. The nodule is real but is it benign? Identification of coarse or complete calcification of the nodule or fat within the nodule is a good indicator of a benign aetiology. In the past, plain film tomography would have been used but now CT scanning is the technique of choice. Ideally, a limited scan through the nodule should be performed with thin sections obtained (1–1.25 mm) using a standard reconstruction algorithm. If the nodule is shown to contain significant calcification or fat then no follow up is required.

3. Nodules identified on CXR are usually 1 cm or greater and, in the absence of any benign features, are likely to require resection. Smaller nodules should be followed up on CT at an interval allowing significant growth to be identified as soon as possible. Typically 3–6 months is the minimum delay to follow up, but a CXR half-way between the original CT and the follow up CT is advisable to detect the rare very rapidly growing tumours.

08 Pneumonias

Pneumonia is a generic term for inflammation within the lung and does not always have an infective aetiology. The characteristic CXR pattern is that of consolidation which may be accompanied by or preceded by ground glass opacification.

Air space filling with pus is the hallmark of bacterial pneumonias; viral pneumonias tend to cause a more interstitial pattern and predominantly ground glass opacification. Clues to the possible causative organisms can be gleaned from the distribution of consolidation and associated features.

8.1 Pulmonary tuberculosis

Pulmonary tuberculosis is caused by *M. tuberculosis*. The host response to TB is dependent on whether the immune system is naïve to the organism and the degree of immunocompetence. Initial infection tends to cause consolidation with spread to regional lymph nodes and subsequent scarring with calcification of the lymph nodes and lung parenchyma; cavitation, if seen, tends to occur later in the infection as the immune response accelerates. Untreated TB becomes dormant and reactivates at times when immune competence is reduced; the immune system is no longer naïve to

the TB organism and mounts an aggressive local response, often resulting in cavitation. TB infection limited to the lung causes consolidation, cavitation, nodularity due to endobronchial plugging and/or granulomas, lymphadenopathy, empyema, and even pneumothorax. Vascular dissemination of TB may occur, with or without clinical lung parenchymal disease, and can result in the infection of any part of the body, causing osteomyelitis, abscesses, meningitis, arthopathy, etc. Involvement of the lung following vascular dissemination results in miliary TB: multiple diffuse small nodules of uniform size, measuring between 1 and 5 mm, scattered throughout the lung, often visible on CXR, but only at around 1 month into the disease.

8.1.1 Inactive pulmonary TB

As stated above, pulmonary TB occasionally resolves spontaneously and enters a latent phase. The manifestations of previous TB infection (see *Fig. 8.1*) on a CXR are typically found in the upper zones and comprise fibrosis, possibly with cavitation and/or traction dilatation of the bronchi, calcified granulomata, and calcified mediastinal/hilar lymph nodes.

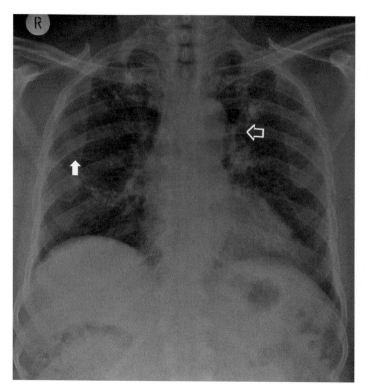

Figure 8.1. Frontal CXR of an adult who had had TB in the past.

Note the calcified nodules and fibrosis in both apices. The left hilum is elevated (open white arrow) as is the minor fissure (white arrow).

8.1.2 Active pulmonary TB

The indicators of active pulmonary TB on a CXR are:
- multifocal consolidation with or without cavitation (*Fig. 8.2*)
- pneumothorax (*Fig. 8.3*)
- unilateral pleural effusion (*Fig. 8.4*)
- new cavity formation (*Fig. 8.5*)
- development of consolidation or nodularity in relation to pre-existing signs of previous TB infection (*Fig. 8.6*)
- thickening of the wall of an existing cavity (*Fig. 8.6*)

None of these findings are specific but if present should prompt investigations targeted at diagnosing TB. A common sequel to resolved pulmonary TB is fibrotic scarring (*Fig. 8.7*), although TB infection may resolve without complication (*Fig. 8.8*).

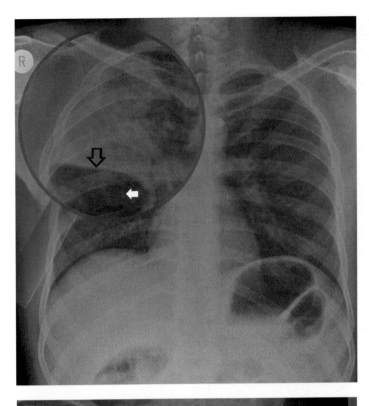

Figure 8.2. Frontal CXR of an adult with pulmonary TB.

Note the right upper lobe consolidation demarcated inferiorly by the horizontal fissure (open black arrow) and the nodularity below the fissure (white arrow) indicating spread to other lobes.

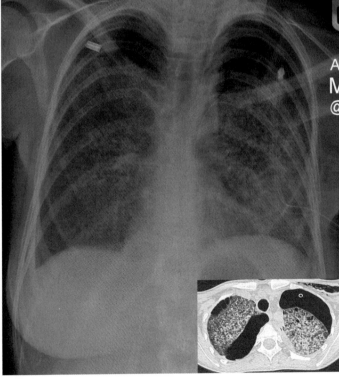

Figure 8.3. Frontal CXR and inset CT image of an adult with pulmonary TB.

The person presented with acute shortness of breath due to bilateral pneumothoraces; a chest drain has been inserted on the left.

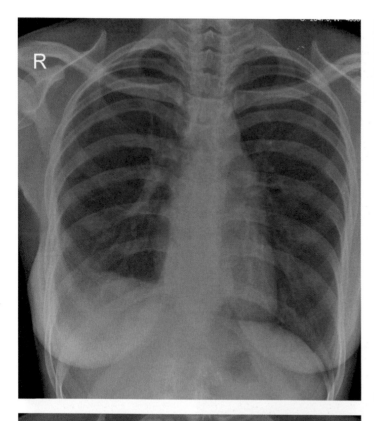

Figure 8.4. Frontal CXR of a young adult with pulmonary TB.

(a) The TB manifest in the lungs as a unilateral pleural effusion. (b) This patient also had back pain and just discernable on the CXR is the discitis at the T11 / T12 level.

(a)

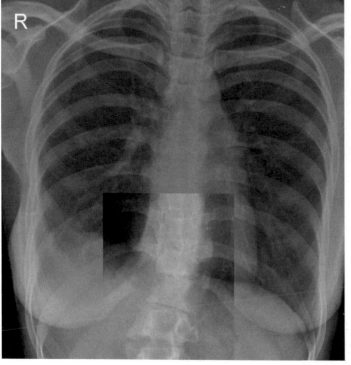

(b)

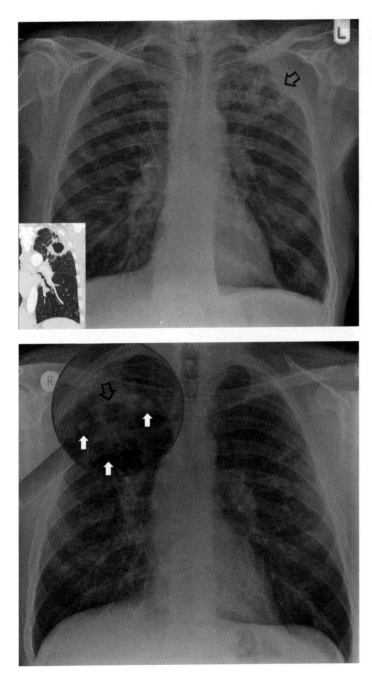

Figure 8.5. Frontal CXR and coronal CT reconstruction inset of an adult with pulmonary TB.

Note the thick-walled cavity in the LUL. In this case this a new cavity with TB identified on bronchial washings.

Figure 8.6. Frontal CXR of an adult with re-activation of TB.

A pre-existing cavity in a region of fibrotic scarring has become thick-walled (open black arrow) and is now associated with nodularity (white arrows), suggesting endobronchial spread of disease. TB was cultured from the sputum.

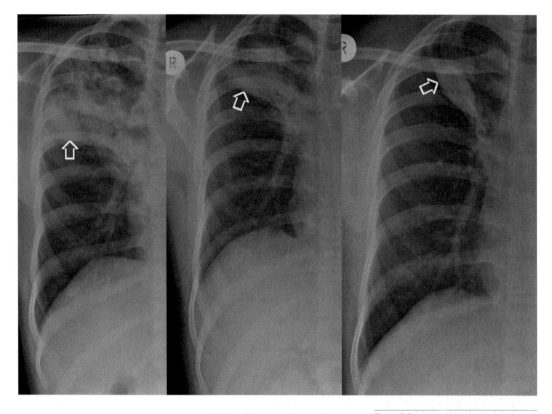

Figure 8.7. A series of images demonstrating the resolution of right upper lobe consolidation due to pulmonary TB during treatment.

Note the elevation of the minor fissure (open white arrow) as the healing process results in fibrous scarring.

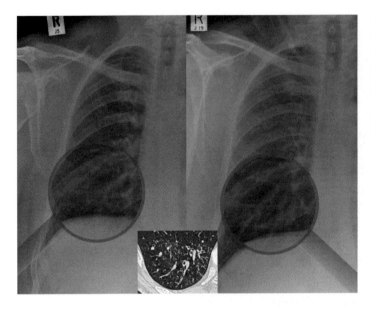

Figure 8.8. Two images from frontal CXRs with an axial CT inset of the same adult.

The left-hand image demonstrates nodularity in the right lower zone when compared to the right-hand image following treatment for TB. The inset image is from a CT at the time of diagnosis and explains that the nodularity seen on the CXR is due to plugging of the distal airways: a typical 'tree in bud' pattern.

8.1.3 Miliary TB

Miliary TB results from the haematogenous spread of the TB infection affecting the entirety of both lungs, with small 1–5 mm soft tissue nodules (*Fig. 8.9*). These only become apparent 1 month into the disease.

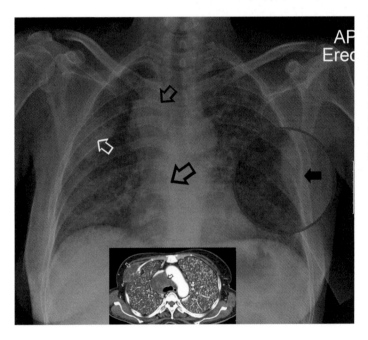

Figure 8.9. Frontal CXR and inset axial CT image of an adult with miliary TB.

Note the diffuse small nodules throughout the lungs. The axial CT inset has a combination of lung parenchymal window and mediastinal window so that the nodularity of the lung parenchyma is seen in conjunction with the mediastinal adenopathy (open black arrow) and rib osteomyelitis (open white arrow). In addition, there is further osteomyelitis and a pathological fracture on the left (black arrow).

8.1.4 TB empyema

Empyema secondary to TB can prove difficult to treat and has a predilection for extending outside the confines of the pleural space and into the chest wall. Even after appropriate treatment the patient may be left with dense pleural calcification (*Fig. 8.10*).

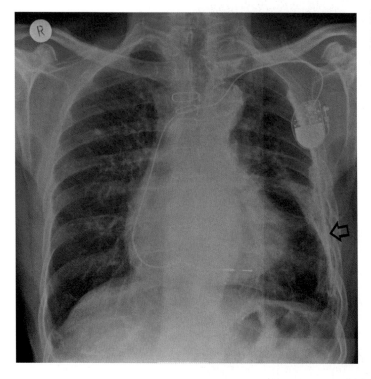

Figure 8.10. Frontal CXR of an adult with a permanent pacemaker.

The dense pleural calcification (open black arrow) was the result of a previous TB empyema.

8.2 Pneumococcal pneumonia

Pneumococcal pneumonia, caused by *Streptococcus pneumoniae*, tends to gives rise to solitary lobar or segmental consolidation (*Fig. 8.11*).

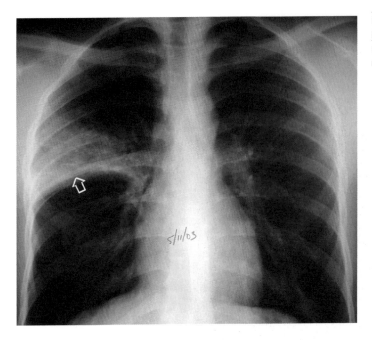

Figure 8.11. Frontal CXR of an adult male with RUL pneumonia.

Note the well defined inferior border formed by the minor fissure (open white arrow).

8.3 Staphylococcal pneumonia

Staphylococcal pneumonia (*Fig. 8.12*) does not tend to be restricted to segments or lobe, it may be multifocal, and it is characteristically associated with cavitation and suppurative changes, causing bulging of the fissures or causing empyemas.

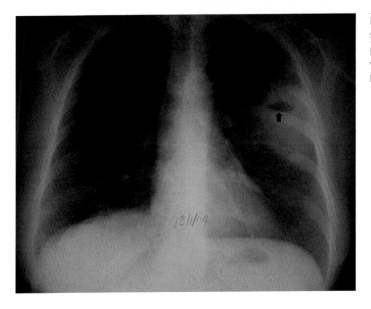

Figure 8.12. Frontal CXR of an adult patient with symptoms of infection.

Note the cavitating pneumonia in the left mid zone with an air–fluid level (black arrow) indicating the presence of an abscess.

A long-term sequel of *Staphylococcus aureus* infection are pneumatoceles. The appearance is similar to that of a cavity but they are thin-walled with no adjacent lung parenchymal opacity to suggest active inflammation (*Fig. 8.13*).

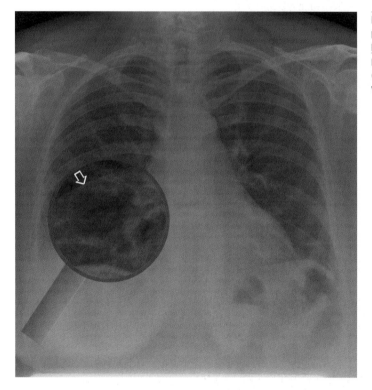

Figure 8.13. This patient had had a staphylococcal pneumonia as a child and has been left with a pneumatocele.

Note that the entirety of the thin wall is visible (open white arrow), unlike the walls of a bulla which appear as isolated curvilinear lines.

8.4 Klebsiella pneumonia

Klebsiella aeruginosa causes a similar pneumonia to staphylococcus. It favours the upper lobes, has a destructive inflammation, with bulging of fissures, abcess formation and subsequent cavitation through to fibrous resolution, similar to pulmonary TB (*Fig. 8.14*).

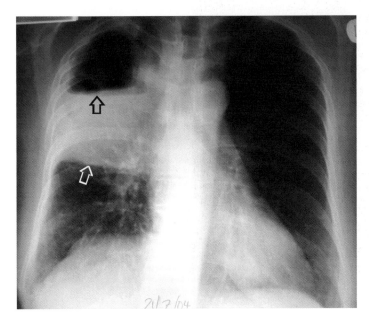

Figure 8.14. Frontal CXR of an adult female with klebsiella pneumonia.

There is a large abscess within the RUL as evidenced by the presence of an air–fluid level (open black arrow) and bulging of the horizontal fissure (open white arrow).

8.5 Eosinophilic pneumonia

The consolidation found in eosinophylic pneumonia results from the accumulation of eosinophil-rich material in the air spaces. Classically, the consolidation 'flits' from site to site with new areas arising as others are resolving spontaneously (*Fig. 8.15*). There are numerous documented causes of eosinophilic pneumonia from drug reactions to parasites (e.g. Loeffler's syndrome), but the cause may not be identified.

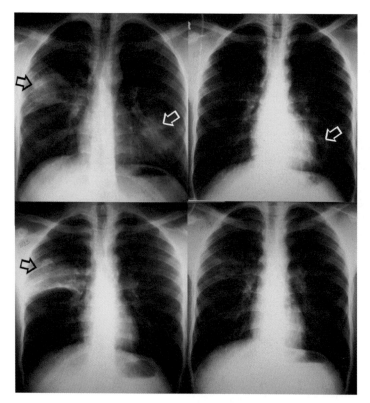

Figure 8.15. A sequence of four CXRs of a patient with eosinophilic pneumonia taken over a period of 18 months.

The sequence is clockwise, starting top left. Note the flitting consolidation in the right upper lobe (open black arrow) and the lingula (open white arrow).

8.6 Opportunistic infections

Organisms that are usually unable to cause pathology in humans may become pathogenic when the immune system is compromised, or there are areas in the body where the immune response is sub-optimal, e.g. cavities. Examples of such opportunistic infections are pneumocystis jiroveci pneumonia (*Fig. 8.16*; previously known as pneumocystis carinii pneumonia) found in immunosuppressed patients, and fungal infections such as aspergillus either in immunosuppressed patients or colonising a cavity (*Fig. 8.17*).

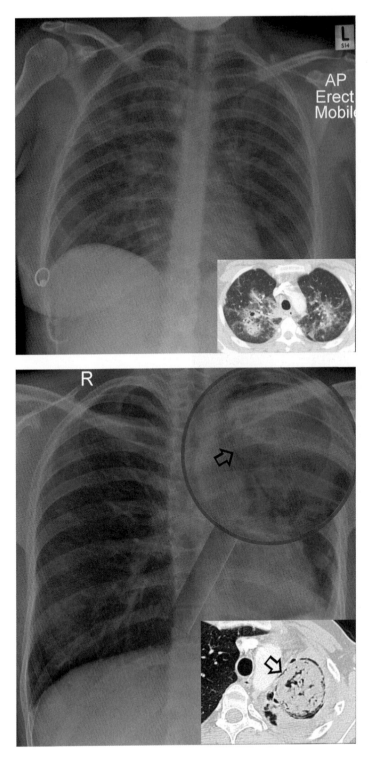

Figure 8.16. Frontal CXR of an immunocompromised adult.

Note the bilateral ground glass opacity tending toward consolidation. On CXR the findings are non-specific and the diagnosis depends on clinical likelihood and microbiological investigation. In this case pneumocystis infection was confirmed on bronchial washings. The air cyst seen on the CT favours pneumocystis infection.

Figure 8.17. Frontal CXR with CT inset of a patient with a mycetoma.

This is a fungal ball, in this case due to aspergillus, that forms following colonisation of a pre-existing lung cavity. Note the 'air-crescent' sign (open black arrow) where the fungal ball fails to reach the inner wall of the cavity, leaving an air space seen as a crescent on CXR.

09 Chronic airways disease

9.1 Asthma

Most asthmatics have a normal CXR – a few have large volume lungs. Asthmatics are prone to spontaneous pneumothorax, pneumomediastinum (*Fig. 9.1*), and mucous plugging which may cause lung opacification and collapse (*Fig. 9.2*).

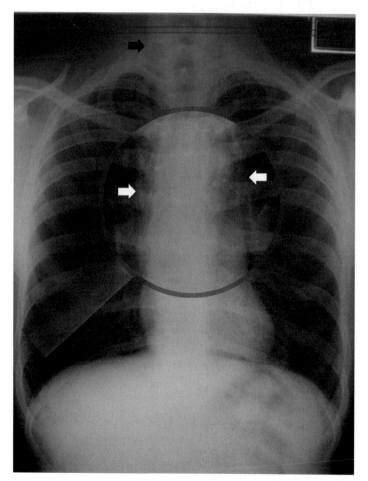

Figure 9.1. Frontal CXR of an adult asthmatic who presented with sudden onset chest pain and dyspnoea.

Note in the magnified area the lucent lines (white arrows) indicating the presence of mediastinal air.

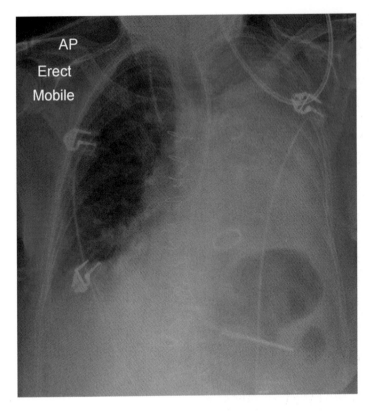

AP

Erect

Mobile

Figure 9.2. Frontal CXR of an asthmatic patient who had recently undergone cardiac surgery.

Day 4 post-op. the patient had rapidly reducing oxygen saturation and an increase in bronchial secretions. Note on the CXR the complete opacification of the left hemithorax, but this is not due to an effusion as there is also significant volume loss causing the mediastinum to shift to the left; this indicates that the underlying pathology is lung collapse. Rapid resolution occurred after aspiration of a large mucous plug in the left main bronchus.

9.2 Chronic bronchitis

Chronic bronchitis is a disease of the airways associated with tobacco smoking (*Fig. 9.3*). Clinical symptoms usually precede any CXR signs, but the accompanying bronchial wall thickening causes the bronchovascular markings to be more prominent on the CXR and perceived further from the hila. Only the proximal bronchi are normally seen on a CXR, but in the outer two-thirds of the lungs only the vessels are visible as the bronchial walls are too thin; in bronchitis the visibility of these more peripheral airways increases the amount of lung markings.

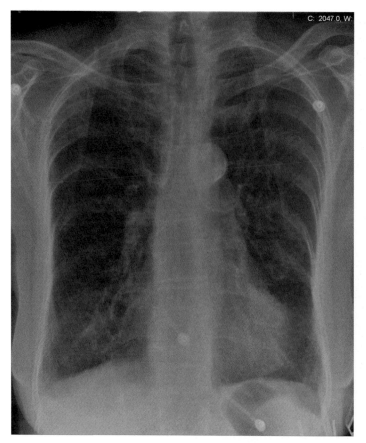

Figure 9.3. Frontal CXR of a long term smoker.

Note the large volume lungs and flattened hemi-diaphragms indicating that this patient probably has underlying emphysema. In addition, there is an overall prominence of the bronchovascular markings; the terms 'dirty' or 'busy' lung, are to be avoided.

9.3 Emphysema

Emphysema is the pathological irreversible destruction of lung tissue, generating areas of lung that do not allow air exchange and are functionally ineffective. The patterns of emphysema are divided into four main types: centrilobular, paraseptal, panacinar and bullous, but considerable overlap exists.

Centrilobular and paraseptal emphysema are not readily identified on CXR unless there is a resultant over-inflation of the lungs. The emphysema must be quite severe for the change in density of the lungs and the degree of change in vascularity to be appreciated on CXR (*Fig. 9.4*). Bullous emphysema, on the other hand, are more readily discernable on CXR because the bullae generate areas on the CXR where there is an obvious paucity of lung markings and the margins of the bullae generate fine curvilinear lines; note that the entirety of the bulla is not seen, only a part of its wall (*Fig. 9.5*). As the commonest cause of emphysema is tobacco smoking, it is not surprising that the disease process tends to be more marked in the better ventilated upper and mid zones; this is at odds with the characteristically basal distribution of panacinar emphysema associated with alpha-1 antitrypsin deficiency. Panacinar emphysema is accompanied by a degree of diminished vascularity that may be readily appreciated on a CXR because there is more lung and therefore more vessels in the lower zones. The diaphragms are usually flattened and vascular shunting to the mid and upper zones can generate an increase in the vascularity of the upper and mid zones that may be erroneously identified as pathological.

The pathological over-expansion of the lungs which occurs in emphysema is assessed by flattening of the hemi-diaphragms. On full inspiration the hemi-diaphragms should retain a domed shape; flattening of this dome is assessed by measuring the maximum perpendicular distance from a line drawn between the cardio and costophrenic angles and the upper surface of the diaphragm.

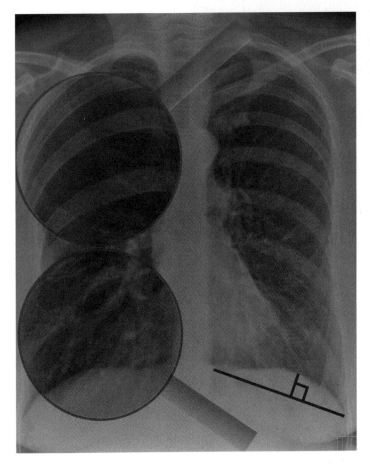

Figure 9.4. Frontal chest radiograph of an adult male smoker.

Note the discrepancy in the vascular markings in the two magnified areas: there are considerably fewer vessels in the upper area as the lung there has been destroyed by emphysema. Note the method of determining whether diaphragmatic flattening is present: a line is imagined connecting the medial and lateral costophrenic angles and the maximum perpendicular height from that line to the hemi-diaphragmatic silhouette should normally be greater than 1.5 cm. Unfortunately, this is a poor negative predictor because normal doming of the diaphragms may be present, as in this case, in spite of extensive emphysema.

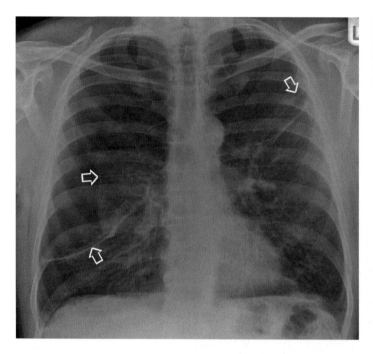

Figure 9.5. Frontal CXR of an adult with severe bullous emphysema.

Note the numerous curvilinear lines (open white arrows) associated with areas of paucity of lung markings where the large bullae are to be found.

9.4 Bronchiectasis

Bronchiectasis is a disease of the airways which manifests as airway dilatation and bronchial wall thickening. Three main types are described: cylindrical, cystic and varicose, but these can be very difficult to appreciate on CXR. The majority of the airways beyond the lobar bronchi are not readily seen on CXR as their walls are too thin; bronchiectatic wall thickening will make airways initially visible more prominent and airways not previously seen will become visible. The first impact this has on the CXR is an impression of an increase in bronchovascular markings similar to chronic bronchitis. In order to identify the airway dilatation component, one has to discern bronchi of larger calibre outside the inner third of the lung, where they would not normally be visible. Classically on CXR, these dilated airways may be appreciated when orientated end-on to the incident X-rays causing ring shadows, or orthogonal to the incident X-rays creating tram-lines (*Fig. 9.6*).

In cylindrical bronchiectasis, the degree of bronchial dilatation is less marked than in the other two forms and the airways are non-tapering but of a generally uniform increase in calibre. The distribution of cylindrical bronchiectasis is usually mid and lower zones and it is associated with immunoglobulin deficiencies and other causes of recurrent infections.

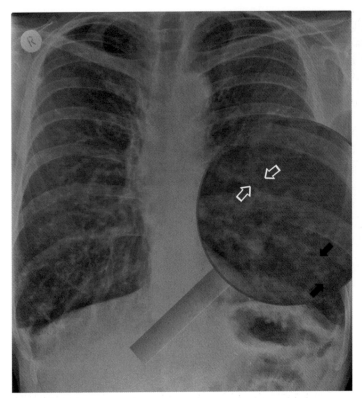

Figure 9.6. Frontal chest radiograph of an adult with severe bronchiectasis.

Note the tram-lines (open white arrows) and ring shadows (black arrows) marked in the magnified area. Now look at the rest of the CXR and see if you can identify the same features elsewhere.

Cystic bronchiectasis produces rings on the CXR but the non-tapering that leads to tram-lining is not a feature. The involved airways demonstrate localised cystic-like dilatation, sometimes dramatic, and the aetiology of this condition is usually post-infective (*Figs 9.7* and *9.8*) or due to chronic mucous plugging as found in cystic fibrosis (*Fig. 9.9*).

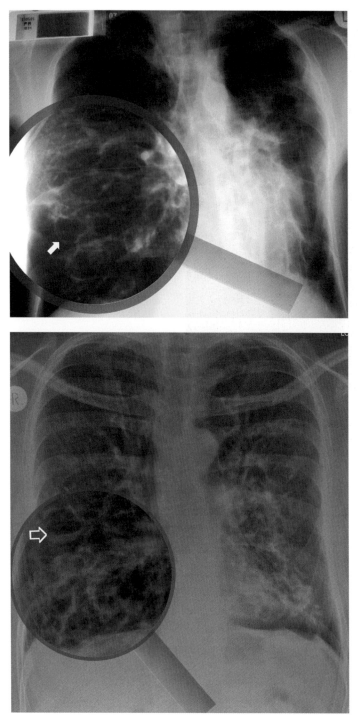

Figure 9.7. Frontal CXR of an adult patient with cystic bronchiectasis.

Note the large thin-walled ring shadows (white arrow) in the magnified area.

Figure 9.8. Frontal CXR of an adult with cystic bronchiectasis in the mid and lower zones.

The ring shadows are thicker walled than in *Figure 9.7* and there are fluid levels (open white arrow) suggesting ongoing infection. Bronchiectatic lung is vulnerable to recurrent infection and colonisation.

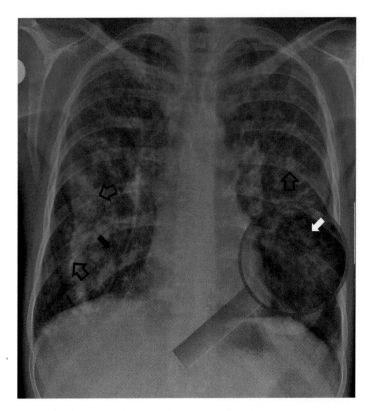

Figure 9.9. Frontal CXR of an adult with cystic fibrosis.

There are bilateral bronchiectatic changes with ring shadows (white arrow) and tram-lines (black arrow). There are bilateral patchy areas of opacification caused by airway plugging and consolidation (open black arrow).

Varicose bronchiectasis describes the airway abnormality that accompanies aspergillus sensitivity in asthmatics: allergic broncho-pulmonary aspergillosis. The distribution is typically mid and upper zones, predominantly central, and the dilatation of the airway is chaotic with discrete regions of markedly dilated airway bounded by normal calibre airway. On CXR, ring shadows may be appreciated, tram-lining is less of a feature, and secondary recurrent flitting consolidation is a strong ancillary sign.

10 Diffuse lung disease

10.1 Interstitial disease – the reticular pattern

The advent of high resolution computed tomography (HRCT) has enabled the identification and classification of numerous diffuse lung diseases. CXR is insensitive at detecting interstitial lung disease, with significant amounts of interstitium effectively 'hidden' on CXR both posteriorly and inferiorly. When the interstitial disease becomes extensive enough to interfere with the clarity of the bronchovascular markings, and occurs more anteriorly such that the clarity of the cardiac silhouette and hemi-diaphragms becomes affected, it can be readily identified on CXR; but determining whether or not this is due to a fibrotic process may still be unclear.

The interstitium is not normally visible on a CXR, but when thickened the interstitium manifests as multiple criss-crossing lines like a net (a process termed reticulation). This process becomes more apparent when the interstitium adjacent to soft tissue structures is involved. The silhouettes seen on the CXR are reliant on the adjacent aerated lung. Reticulation along the border between interstitium and aerated lung produces a fine irregularity to the interface, making it less clearly defined and so obscuring the silhouette (this is termed the interface sign). This affects the clarity of the bronchovascular markings as well as the pleural and mediastinal silhouettes.

In the presence of reticulation, caution should be taken when identifying co-existent nodules because the overlaying of multiple net-like patterns will mimic nodules at the cross-over points. The addition of nodularity in the presence of reticulation really does assist the diagnostic process in any case.

10.1.1 Interstitial fibrosis

Clues on a CXR to implicate fibrosis as the cause for a reticular pattern are:
- loss of volume either globally or locally (*Figs 10.1* and *10.2*)
- distortion of the lung architecture
- the presence of traction dilatation of the airways, which may result in ring shadows
- the presence of honeycomb destruction which, when severe, may be apparent on CXR (*Fig. 10.3*)

The final interpretation often relies heavily on the clinical history and exclusion of non-fibrotic causes of reticulation. Note that in the presence of co-existent emphysema (see *Fig. 10.2*) the lung volumes may be normal and this should not be used as a criterion to exclude pulmonary fibrosis.

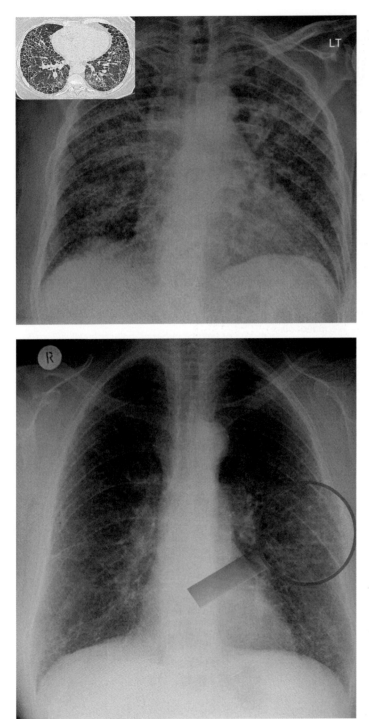

Figure 10.1. Frontal CXR and axial CT inset of an adult with advanced idiopathic pulmonary fibrosis.

The coarse reticular pattern is primarily due to honeycomb destruction, but there is also a significant amount of interstitial fibrosis contributing to the extensive reticulation.

Figure 10.2. Frontal CXR of an adult with co-existent emphysema and idiopathic pulmonary fibrosis.

Note the reticulation extending into the mid zones, but normal volume lungs.

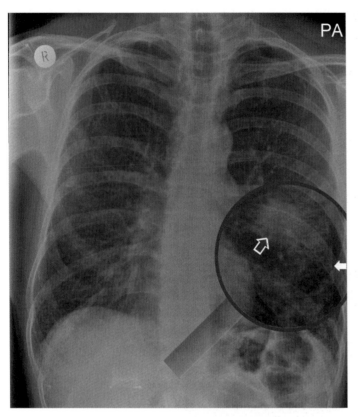

PA

Figure 10.3. Frontal CXR of an adult male with a primary lung carcinoma (open white arrow).

This is a post-biopsy film, hence the pneumothorax making the sub-pleural honeycomb destruction at the lung edge (white arrow) easier to see.

10.1.2 Lymphangitis carcinomatosa

Lymphangitis carcinomatosa is the descriptive term for infiltration of the lymphatic vessels by a tumour, resulting in interstitial thickening. The thickening is due to the cellular infiltrate itself and also the result of lymphatic congestion causing fluid retention. Bearing this in mind, a large tumour may physically obstruct the lymphatic system causing a lymphangitic picture without true tumour invasion. The distinction is not usually discernable even on CT scanning and requires a judgment call at a multidisciplinary meeting to decide how best to proceed.

On CXR, the main appearance is that of reticulation. As there is a lymphatic congestion component, some degree of ground glass opacification is likely and septal lines tend to be a prominent feature. All these features can be found in heart failure but, when unilateral, heart failure is less likely (see *Fig. 7.8*).

10.2 LAM

Lymphangioleiomyomatosis (LAM) is a rare disease found in women and which has a very poor prognosis. Histologically, LAM is identical to tuberous sclerosis in the lungs, forming multiple small thin-walled air cysts throughout the lung with no zonal preference. On HRCT these cysts are readily identified, but on CXR the overriding pattern is an apparent reticulation; the multiple small 'holes' are mistaken for the normal lung and the walls and intervening normal lung are taken to be the interstitium. The clue to the true nature of the pattern is the absence of the interface sign. An extensive interstitial pattern should obscure the silhouettes on the CXR, but as the cysts in LAM are not sub-pleural in location, the mediastinal silhouettes are preserved and, in the absence of fibrosis, lung volumes are normal (*Fig. 10.4*).

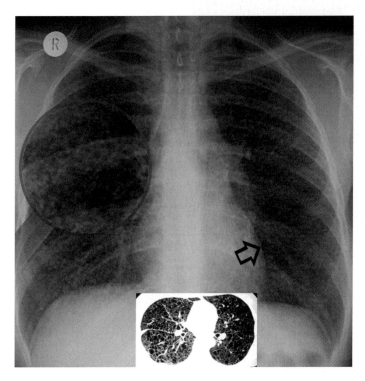

Figure 10.4. Frontal CXR of an adult with lymphangioleiomyomatosis.

Note that the apparent reticulation in the magnified area is actually due to multiple small air-filled cysts (see the HRCT image inset), as these do not have a predilection for the sub-pleural regions; the silhouettes on the CXR are relatively unaffected (open black arrow).

10.3 Langerhans cell histiocytosis

Langerhans cell histiocytosis (LCH) is another cause of diffuse air-filled cysts in the lungs (*Fig. 10.5*). The key to distinguishing LCH from LAM is the distribution. LCH is a disease related to tobacco smoking and has an upper and mid zone distribution akin to smoking-associated centrilobular emphysema. This distribution is apparent through the relative sparing of the bases of the lungs. In addition, LCH begins as a nodular disease with air-filled cysts, due to cavitation of those nodules, and focal bronchial dilatation appearing later as the disease progresses. The presence of nodules would therefore favour LCH over LAM. The distinction is far more straightforward on HRCT and is an important one because LCH may respond well to a cessation of smoking.

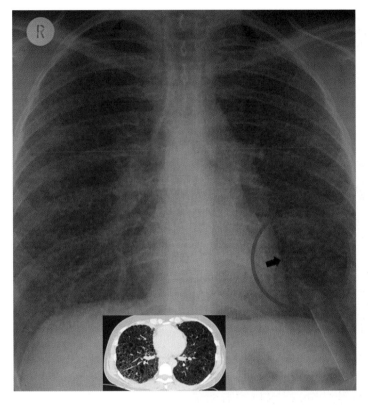

Figure 10.5. Frontal CXR and axial CT inset of an adult with LCH.

At this stage of the LCH, the predominant abnormality is cystic but some nodules remain and, on a CXR, the appearances are difficult to differentiate from interstitial lung disease. The sparing of the sub-pleural region preserving the cardiac (black arrow) and diaphragmatic silhouettes is the clue to the parenchymal site of this abnormality.

10.4 Pulmonary sarcoid

Sarcoidosis is a systemic granulomatous condition and has a deserved reputation for being the greatest mimic in chest radiology. Classically, sarcoidosis manifests in the chest as bilateral hilar and mediastinal adenopathy (*Figs 10.6* and *10.7*), indistinguishable from lymphoma and TB which are the two main differential diagnoses. In general, patients with sarcoid are clinically in better health than their CXR suggests.

When sarcoid involves the lung parenchyma it may form multiple small nodules mimicking miliary TB (*Fig. 10.8*) or metastases, consolidation (often multi-focal) mimicking infections or alveolar cell carcinoma, or large nodules / masses mimicking primary or metastatic malignancies (see *Fig. 7.6*). A histological diagnosis is often required, but the presence of peri-lymphatic nodularity (i.e adjacent to the bronchovascular bundles, interlobular septa and the fissures) identified on HRCT may be sufficient, in the absence of significant symptoms, to settle for sarcoidosis as a diagnosis (*Fig. 10.9*).

Sarcoid in the lungs may progress to fibrosis (*Fig. 10.10*), which tends to be coarse in nature with parenchymal bands and distortion in a mid and upper zone peri-hilar distribution.

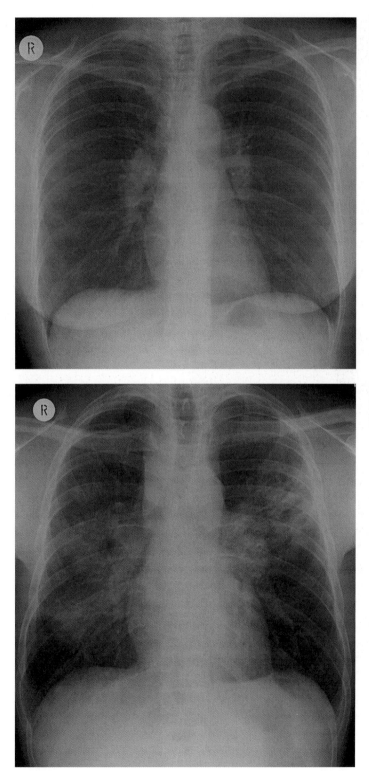

Figure 10.6. Frontal CXR of an adult with sarcoidosis. This is the classic presentation with bilateral hilar adenopathy.

Figure 10.7. Frontal CXR of an adult with sarcoidosis, in this instance presenting as bilateral mid zone consolidation in conjunction with left hilar adenopathy.

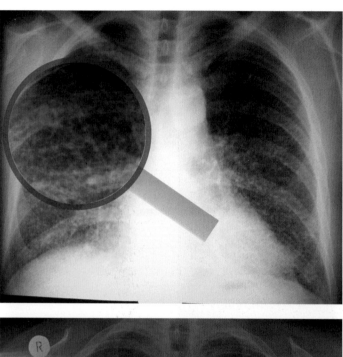

Figure 10.8. Frontal CXR of an adult with sarcoidosis.

Note the numerous small nodules mimicking miliary TB. Clinically this patient was asymptomatic.

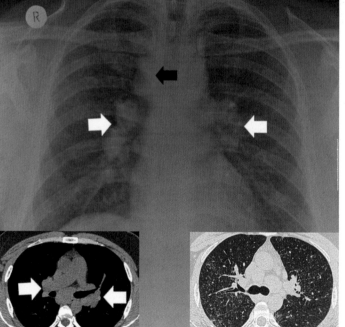

Figure 10.9. Frontal CXR and axial CT insets of an adult with sarcoidosis.

Note the bilateral hilar adenopathy (white arrows), para-tracheal adenopathy (black arrow) and, on the inset CT images, there is sub-carinal adenopathy and fine nodularity, which is less apparent on CXR.

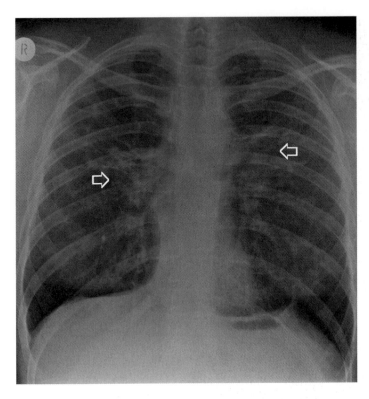

Figure 10.10. Frontal CXR of an adult with burnt out sarcoid.

Note the predominantly mid zone peri-hilar distribution of the fibrosis (open white arrows) causing increased opacification and distortion of the lung. This distribution is typical of sarcoid.

10.5 Hypersensitivity pneumonitis

Hypersensitivity pneumonitis (HP) is caused by inhaled organic allergens causing type 2 and type 4 hypersensitivity reactions, resulting in lung damage. The condition was previously known as extrinsic allergic alveolitis and this term is still in common use. The clinical and radiological manifestations of HP depend upon the timing of the exposure to the allergen.

Acute HP (*Fig. 10.11*) results from acute exposure to the allergen, resulting in a viral-like illness that rarely presents to a doctor as removal from the allergen source is usually sufficient to relieve the symptoms.

Sub-acute HP (*Fig. 10.12*) results from repeated exposure to the allergen; lung function progressively deteriorates and the patient's cough and dyspnoea usually lead to them seeking medical advice. At this stage the main radiology finding is of ill-defined centrilobular nodules and ground glass opacification. The nodules are readily seen on HRCT, but may be difficult to discern on CXR.

A failure to avoid the causative allergen during the sub-acute phase of the disease results in the development of irreversible fibrosis (*Fig. 10.13*), more often to be found in the upper zones.

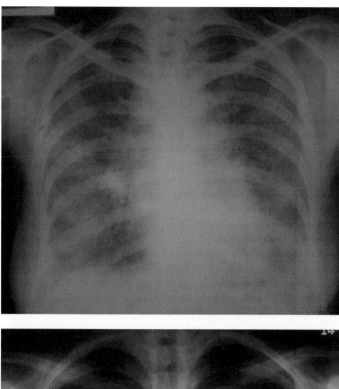

Figure 10.11. Frontal CXR of a patient admitted with acute hypersensitivity pneumonitis.

Appearances are non-specific with bilateral consolidation and the diagnosis was made clinically.

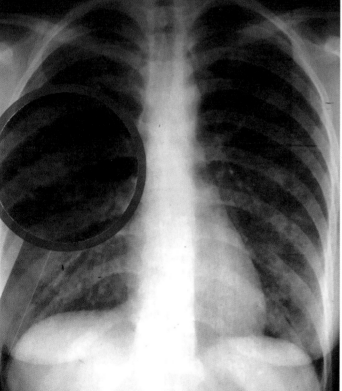

Figure 10.12. Frontal CXR of an adult with sub-acute hypersensitivity pneumonitis.

The changes are subtle, with nodularity just discernable on the CXR.

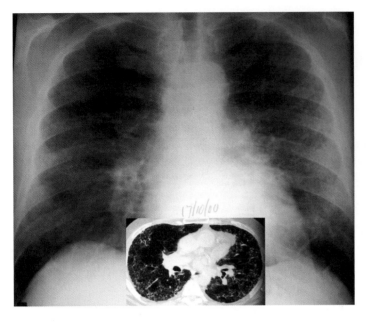

Figure 10.13. Frontal CXR and inset HRCT image of an adult with chronic hypersensitivity pneumonitis.

Note the bilateral mid zone reticulation confirmed on CT to represent fibrosis.

11 Pleural disease

The pleura is one of the simplest and yet most ingenious mechanisms in the body. Inhalation results from an increase in the intra-thoracic volume, causing a negative intra-thoracic pressure, thereby drawing air in. This is achieved by chest expansion in the coronal and sagittal plains by the elevation of the ribs which are effectively hinged at the spine. The foreshortening of the chest that results is offset and reversed by depression of the hemi-diaphragms; as a result the lung must expand to fill a thorax that has changed shape and it can only do this if the surface of the lung is able to slide across the inner surface of the chest wall and yet remain attached to it. The pleura is a thin membrane that may be likened to a sealed 'bag' containing a small amount of fluid that is wrapped around the lung forming two layers, one attached to the lung, the visceral pleura, and one attached to the inside of the chest wall, the parietal pleura. Each lung has its own pleural 'bag'. The surface tension of the thin film of water is 'sticky' enough to keep the two layers of pleura firmly attached and yet allow them to slide over each other.

An understanding of the mechanism of action of the pleura explains the impact that a pneumothorax or pleural effusion may have on lung function.

11.1 Effusion

There is normally a small amount of fluid in the pleural space 'gluing' and 'lubricating' the two layers of pleura. This fluid is constantly being absorbed and generated, and an imbalance in this equilibrium can cause accumulation of fluid in the pleural space, for example, the increased generation and / or reduced absorption of pleural fluid. Heart failure and inflammation of the pleura (pleuritis) are the commonest causes of pleural effusions. In heart failure there is an increase in fluid production due the saturation of the interstitium with fluid. In pleuritis, usually secondary to a pneumonia, there is a seepage of fluid from the inflamed pleura, which in itself is less capable of absorbing that fluid (*Fig. 11.1*).

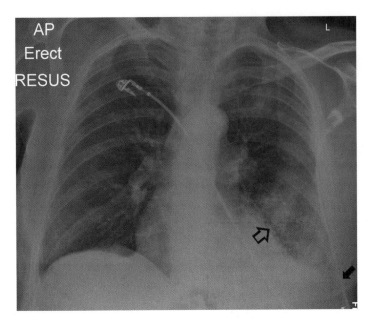

Figure 11.1. AP CXR of an adult with left lower lobe pneumonia and a parapneumonic effusion blunting the left costophrenic angle (black arrow).

Note the left heart border remains clear (open black arrow) indicating that the consolidation is in the lower lobe and not the lingula.

11.1.1 Simple pleural effusion

In a simple pleural effusion, the pleural space is continuous allowing fluid to accumulate anywhere, such that simple effusions tend to accumulate in the dependent areas of the chest. If the patient is imaged in an erect position the fluid accumulates at the bases giving a meniscus like appearance (*Figs 11.2–11.4*). In a supine patient the fluid accumulates in the posterior of the chest and may only manifest as an increase in density. The appearance of an effusion with the patient semi-erect is the hardest to delineate. CXRs taken on the ward are taken with the patient lying in bed, propped up leaning back against the X-ray plate, in effect semi-erect. In order to achieve as close as possible the appearance of a true erect film, the radiographer will angle the X-ray source downwards to compensate for the semi-erect position of the patient; these films are labelled 'AP erect' but would be more accurately labelled 'AP not supine' and the alteration in the orientation of the incident X-rays has a profound effect on the appearance of fluid on the CXR (*Fig. 11.5*). A developing pleural effusion will occupy space in the hemi-thorax, resulting in compensatory collapse of the lung. When the threshold of this accommodation is reached, the pleural effusion will begin to increase the size of the ipsilateral hemithorax at the expense of the contralateral hemi-thorax, causing a shift of the mediastinum away from the effusion (*Fig. 11.6*).

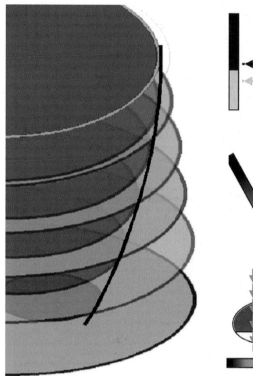

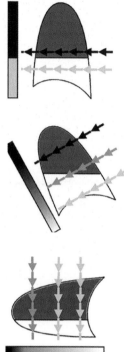

Figure 11.2. Pleural effusion.

The left image explains the meniscus appearance (black line) of a pleural effusion. Note that it is not due to the fluid being loculated in the lateral hemi-thorax, but is a result of the shape of the pleural space being filled; the fluid (light grey) anterior and posterior to the underlying aerated lung (dark grey) has less influence on the overall density of the CXR than the fluid found laterally where there is no aerated lung. The meniscus is formed by the demarcation between the collapsing lung and the pleural fluid. Note that the top of the effusion is at the top of the meniscus. The three images on the right demonstrate how the demarcation of the fluid level becomes less clear-cut as the orientation of the fluid level to the incident X-rays becomes less favourable. The arrows represent the incident X-rays and the shaded bar the resulting density change on the X-ray image.

Figure 11.3. Frontal CXR of an adult with a simple right pleural effusion.

This demonstrates the meniscal appearance described in *Figure 11.2* (black arrow). Note also the difference in density of the lower zones. On the right there is fluid in front of and behind the aerated lung, increasing the density but not obscuring the vessels.

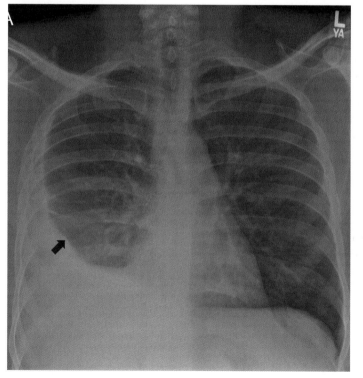

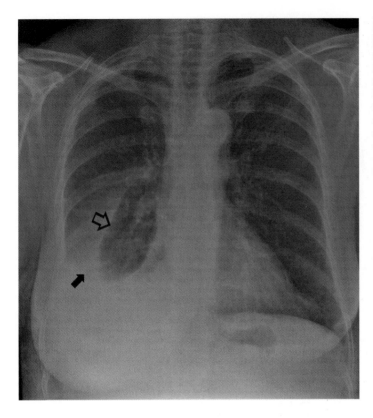

Figure 11.4. Frontal CXR of an adult female with a large unilateral pleural effusion.

Note the typical meniscus sign (black arrow), but also a further line curving upward and medially, crossing the minor fissure (open black arrow). This is fluid tracking into the major fissure, but not loculated as in a later example *(Fig. 12.11)*. A unilateral pleural effusion is a concerning finding and in this case, where there is evidence of breast surgery (note the asymmetry in the breast shadows), recurrent breast carcinoma is a likely cause.

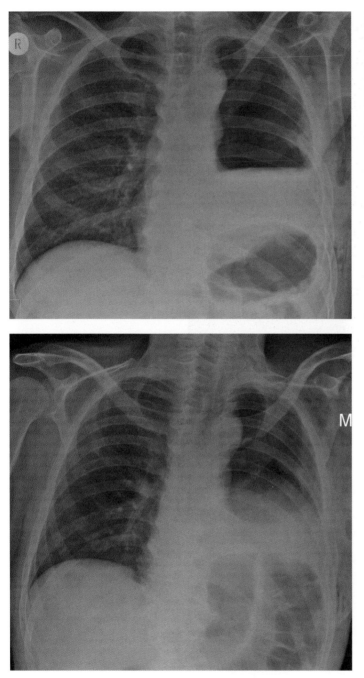

(a)

(b)

Figure 11.5. Frontal CXR of an adult following a left pneumonectomy.

(a) As is normal, the hemithorax is filling with fluid and on this erect film the air–fluid level is readily identified. In (b), the CXR was taken AP with the patient semi-erect. The orientation of the clavicles matches that in (a) so the X-rays have been angled down; as a result, the air–fluid level is no longer orientated in line with the X-rays and therefore is replaced by a graded change in density.

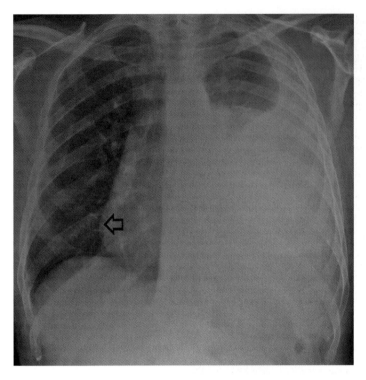

Figure 11.6. Frontal CXR of an adult with a large left-sided pleural effusion.

Note the mediastinal displacement to the right (open black arrow).

When the patient is supine the fluid accumulates posteriorly causing a general increase in density on the CXR. A margin is only revealed if there is sufficient fluid to displace the lung from the lateral chest wall, at which point the presence of fluid becomes more obvious (*Figs 11.7* and *11.8*).

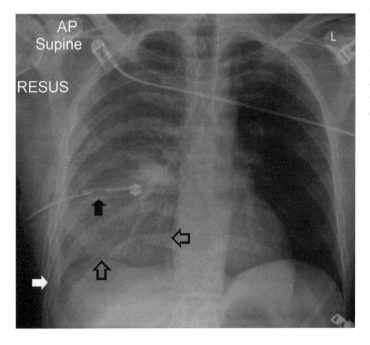

Figure 11.7. Supine CXR of an adult male with a large right-sided traumatic haemothorax.

Note the fluid tracking up the side separating the lung from the chest wall (white arrow), and the preservation of the diaphragmatic silhouette and the right heart border (open black arrows) as the fluid lies posteriorly. This patient has a chest drain *in situ* with a side hole (black arrow).

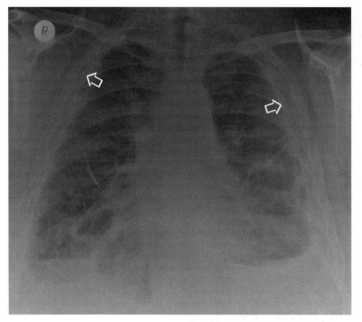

Figure 11.8. Supine CXR of an adult male.

There are bilateral pleural effusions making distinction by transradiancy difficult, but note the tracking of the fluid laterally pushing the lung away from the chest wall (open white arrow).

With the patient semi-erect (*Fig. 11.9*), as is usually the case for portable ward-based CXRs, the CXR only reveals some increased density in the lower region of the chest. The fluid will tend to lie posteriorly and may therefore fail to occupy the lateral costophrenic angle or obscure the hemi-diaphragmatic silhouette; a clear costophrenic angle is often taken as an indication that there is no pleural fluid, but this would be erroneous in such a situation.

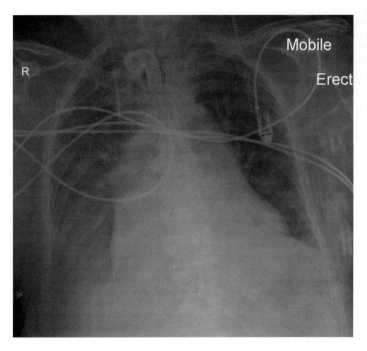

Figure 11.9. AP semi-erect CXR of an adult with a large right pleural effusion.

There is no meniscus due to the orientation of the patient and compensating downward angulation of the incident X-rays (see *Fig. 11.2*). Note the right heart border and medial right hemi-diaphragmatic silhouettes are spared as the fluid lies posteriorly in the chest.

11.1.2 Sub-pulmonic pleural effusion

Sometimes with the patient erect, pleural fluid collects between the inferior surface of the lung and the hemi-diaphragm (*Fig. 11.10*). It is not trapped there and will flow into the posterior hemithorax when the patient is supine, but on a frontal CXR it may be difficult to identify. The preservation of the inferior contour of the aerated lung generates the appearance of a diaphragmatic silhouette and a clear costophrenic angle, when in actuality the diaphragm itself is more inferior. Clues to the presence of a sub-pulmonic effusion are apparent elevation of the hemi-diaphragm, displacement of the fundus of the stomach from the apparent left diaphragmatic surface, lateral peaking of the apparent diaphragmatic silhouette, and a loss of the contour when the CXR is taken supine.

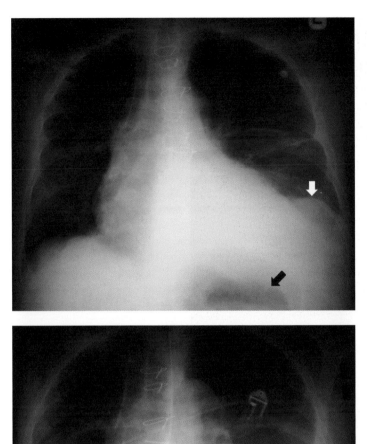

Figure 11.10. Frontal (a) erect and (b) semi-erect CXRs of an adult with a sub-pulmonic pleural effusion.

(a) Note that there is apparently a clear costophrenic angle, the fluid has collected under the lung; the clue to this is the lateral peaking of the apparent hemi-diaphragm (white arrow), more usually central or medial, and the distance between this and the gastric fundus (black arrow).
(b) When the patient is semi-erect, the fluid escapes posteriorly causing increased lower zone opacification but preserving the left heart border (black arrow).

(a)

(b)

11.1.3 Complex pleural effusion

A convex or straight contour to a pleural effusion indicates some degree of complexity, either due to increased viscosity of the fluid so that it is not free-flowing, or enclosure within a restricted space, i.e. loculated due to fibrous septa or tethered lung. The fluid is not free to travel to dependent areas and therefore behaves very differently to a simple pleural effusion. Complexity in a pleural effusion suggests haemothorax or empyema (*Fig. 11.11*) but may be the chronic sequel of an unresolved simple effusion.

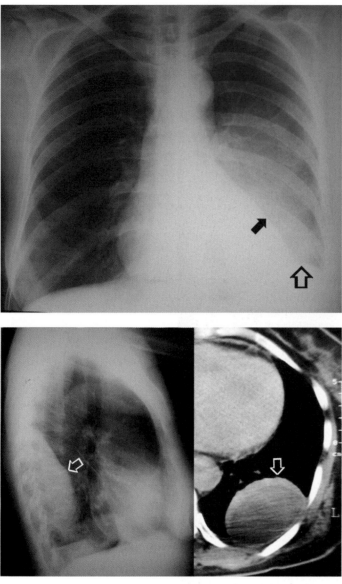

(a)

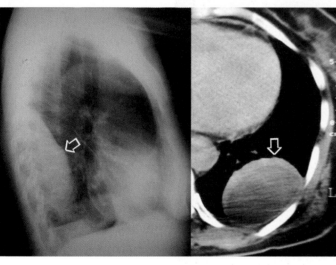

(b)

Figure 11.11. Empyema in an adult.

(a) Frontal erect CXR of an adult with a posteriorly loculated empyema. If this were a simple pleural effusion, the left heart border (black arrow) and left hemi-diaphragm (open black arrow) would be obscured.

(b) Lateral CXR and part of the CT scan of the same patient demonstrating the posterior location of this pleural collection. The anterior margin of the empyema is marked (open white arrow), and convexity in the margins of pleural fluid favour empyema as the cause.

Empyema is an important diagnosis to make as it rarely resolves without some form of drainage and can extend into the lung forming abscesses and reach outside the thorax. TB empyema in particular has a tendency to extrude through the thoracic cage and diaphragm (*Fig. 11.12*). Note that in the early stages an infected pleural effusion may be simple rather than complex in appearance.

Percutaneous drainage should be attempted prior to surgical drainage and there is *anecdotal* evidence to suggest fibrinolytic agents may improve the effectiveness of drainage of complex collections by breaking down the septations. Once an empyema has been resolved there may be residual pleural thickening; a baseline CXR at that stage is of use when attempting to identify new pathology on subsequent CXRs. The long-term sequel of either an empyema (particularly TB) or a haemothorax may be extensive pleural calcification (see *Fig. 11.28*).

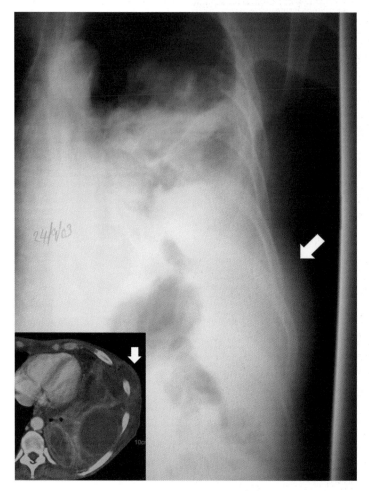

Figure 11.12. Part of a frontal CXR and inset axial CT image of an adult with TB empyema.

The contour of the chest wall reveals extrusion of the empyema into the chest wall tissues (white arrow).

Simple pleural effusions may form locules within the fissures forming pseudo-tumours (*Fig. 11.13*). Loculation within the oblique fissures is best appreciated on a lateral CXR (*Fig. 11.14*).

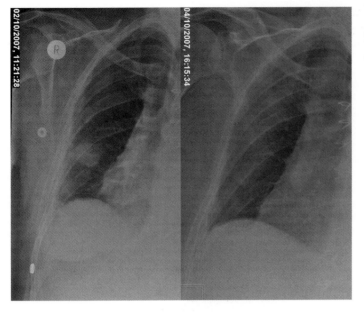

Figure 11.13. Images from two CXRs taken two days apart.

The apparent nodule on the left hand image was due to loculated fluid within the oblique fissure and is no longer visible on the subsequent CXR.

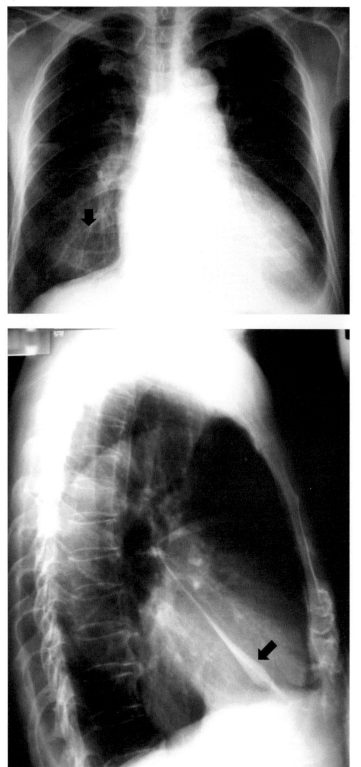

(a)

(b)

Figure 11.14. Comparison of (a) frontal and (b) lateral CXR for a pseudo-tumour.

(a) Frontal CXR of an adult with an area of increased density in the right lower zone (black arrow).
(b) The patient was recalled for a lateral CXR which confirmed the cause to be loculated fluid in the right oblique fissure (black arrow).

11.2 Pneumothorax

A pneumothorax describes the presence of air in the pleural space. In the absence of trauma the source of that air will be the lung or, much more rarely, the tracheo-bronchial tree. People susceptible to spontaneous pneumothorax in the absence of trauma or underlying pathology are tall thin males with 'long' lungs who tend to have small apical sub-pleural blebs that may spontaneously rupture (*Fig. 11.15*). There are many disease processes that predispose to pneumothorax, including obstructive lung disease (including asthma, cystic fibrosis and emphysema), TB, cavitating infections, cavitating metastases (osteosarcoma is a classic example), and some rare disorders like LCH and LAM.

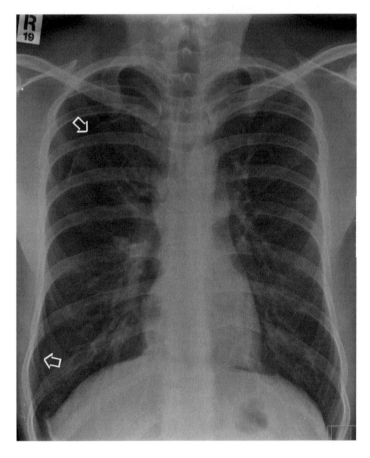

Figure 11.15. Frontal CXR of a tall thin young male who presented with sudden onset left pleuritic chest pain.

The history is highly suggestive of a spontaneous pneumothorax and the blunting of the left costophrenic angle is consistent with that diagnosis; the fluid trapped in the pleural space is able to accumulate in the most dependent area. Careful scrutiny reveals the lung edge (white arrows).

The presence of air in the pleural space detaches the visceral from the parietal pleura, allowing the lung to collapse due to its inherent elasticity (left to its own devices the lung will happily recoil and empty of air – it is this tendency that causes unforced expiration, such that control of unforced expiration is actually through a gradual release of inspiratory effort). The loss of the adhesion between the visceral and parietal pleura decouples the lung from the chest wall, dramatically reducing the efficacy of breathing.

As the lung collapses away from the chest wall in the presence of a pneumothorax, there should be no vascular markings beyond the lung edge (*Fig. 11.16*). Careful scrutiny is required to ensure this is the case as skin folds on the chest, especially on portable CXRs, can mimic a lung edge (a pseudo-pneumothorax). When a CXR is taken on the ward, the X-ray plate is placed behind the patient and the patient sits semi-erect leaning against the plate to hold it in position. The combination of the patient leaning against the plate and the likelihood they have lost some weight in hospital, results in loose skin that has a tendency to 'ruck' in such a way as to mimic a lung edge on CXR (*Fig. 11.17*). The clues to this process are the presence of vessels beyond the lung edge and the inability to follow that apparent lung edge around the thorax as far as one would expect the lung edge, due to a pneumothorax, to extend.

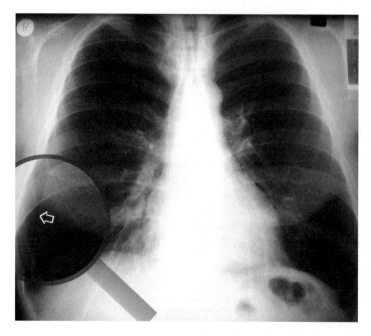

Figure 11.16. Frontal CXR of an adult with a right sided pneumothorax.

The lung edge is marked (open white arrow) and beyond this there are no vascular markings. Compare this appearance to that of *Figure 11.17*.

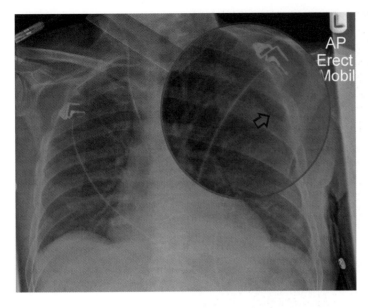

Figure 11.17. AP CXR of an adult with a pseudo-pneumothorax.

In the magnified region there is an apparent lung edge (open black arrow) but beyond this there are clearly lung markings.

A pneumothorax should resolve spontaneously if the source of air is stopped, but the process can be accelerated by aspiration or drainage. If the air leak persists a bronchopleural fistula develops, and only when this fistula closes either spontaneously or following intervention will the pneumothorax resolve. If the air leak causing the pneumothorax only allows air into the pleural space and not out, then a tension pneumothorax develops. In this situation, the intrapleural pressure on the affected side pushes the mediastinum to the opposite side, causing compromise of the mediastinal vasculature and the trachea; this is a critical condition and requires immediate drainage. If, in the presence of a pneumothorax, there is a shift of the mediastinum away from the pneumothorax (*Fig. 11.18*) and / or flattening of the hemi-diaphragm on the affected side (*Figs 11.19* and *11.20*), the presence of a tension pneumothorax should be suspected and the pneumothorax pressure released.

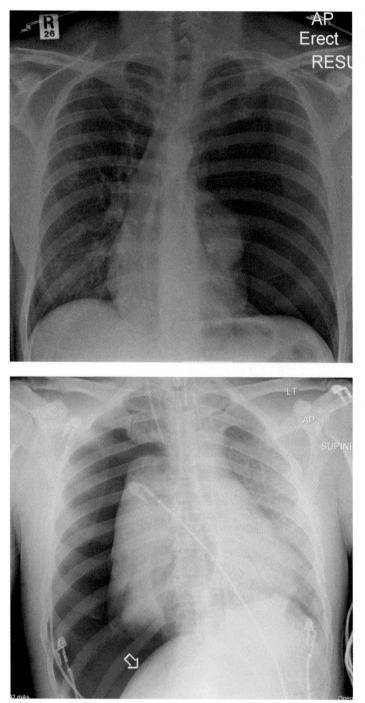

Figure 11.18. AP CXR of an adult with a left pneumothorax.

Note that the left pneumothorax has completely collapsed the left lung and is shifting the mediastinum to the right, indicating the presence of a tension pneumothorax. There is no hemi-diaphragmatic flattening on this CXR.

Figure 11.19. AP CXR of an adult patient with a right-sided tension pneumothorax.

Note the flattening of the right hemi-diaphragm (open white arrow).

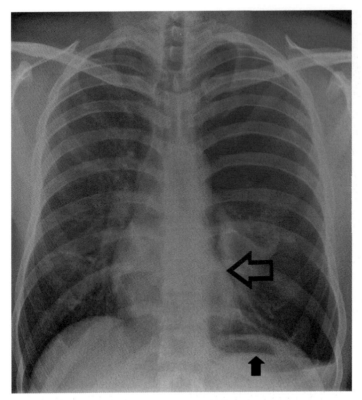

Figure 11.20. Frontal CXR of an adult with a left-sided tension pneumothorax.

Note the mediastinal shift to the right (open black arrow) and the partial flattening of the left hemi-diaphragm (black arrow). Remember that the hemi-diaphragm is a three-dimensional structure and so, in this case, anterior doming conceals posterior flattening.

A pneumothorax may be complicated by the extension of air into the adjacent soft tissues resulting in soft tissue emphysema. In the soft tissues of the lateral chest wall air is readily visible, but the same air in the soft tissues anterior or posterior to the chest may cause some confusion as to the appearance of the underlying lung. Sometimes the air tracks into the pectoralis muscles (*Fig. 11.21*) and is readily identified there. Extension of air into the mediastinum can be more difficult to identify (*Fig. 11.22*) and is sometimes only apparent as a thin lucent line outlining the mediastinal contour (*Fig. 11.23*).

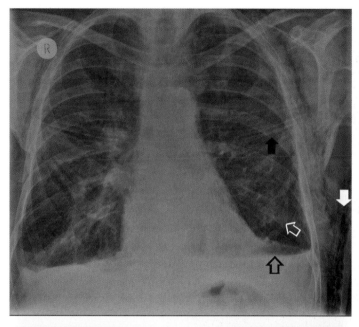

Figure 11.21. AP CXR on an adult following cardiac surgery.

There is a left-sided hydropneumothorax – note the lung edge (open white arrow) and the air–fluid level (open black arrow). There is also a right-sided pleural effusion and bilateral chest wall soft tissue emphysema – note the black areas in the sub-cutaneous tissues (white arrow) and the lucent lines radiating from the shoulders (black arrow) caused by air in the pectoralis muscles.

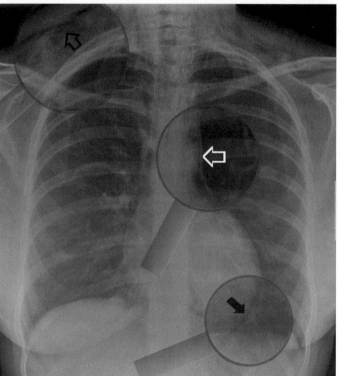

Figure 11.22. AP CXR of an adult with a pneumomediastinum.

Note the soft tissue emphysema on the right (open black arrow) indicating an air leak has occurred. The more subtle signs are the lucencies separating the mediastinum from the pleura at the aortic knuckle (open white arrow) and the left cardiophrenic angle (black arrow), due to free air in the mediastinum.

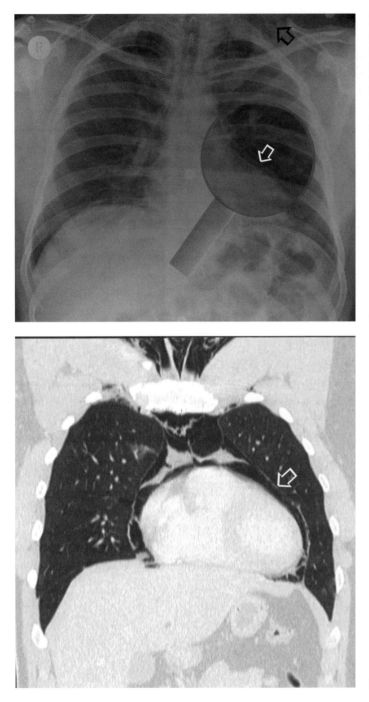

(a)

(b)

Figures 11.23. Traumatic pneumomediastinum in an adult.

(a) AP CXR of an adult with a traumatic pneumomediastinum tracking into the soft tissues of the chest wall (open black arrow). Note the free mediastinal air at the left heart border (open white arrow) demonstrated on (b), a coronal reconstruction from a CT scan.

(c) A coronal reconstruction from a more posterior position, demonstrating further free mediastinal air and the soft tissue emphysema (open black arrow).

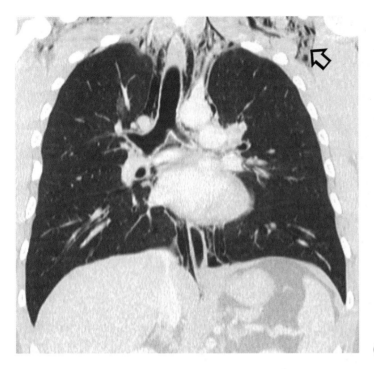

(c)

If the patient is semi-erect or supine, the lung will preferentially occupy the posterior part of the hemithorax leaving the pneumothorax in the anterior part. If the size of the pneumothorax is insufficient to separate the lung from the lateral chest wall, there may not be a lung edge at the correct orientation to form a line on the CXR (*Fig. 11.24*). This leaves only the difference between aerated lung and air as the distinguishing element – a tall order for the contrast resolution of a CXR. Caution should therefore be taken when reading a supine or semi-erect CXR, especially in the context of a suspected pneumothorax. The silhouette formed by free air, as opposed to aerated lung, is sharper, and where aerated lung is displaced by air the difference in density may be perceived; this occurs at the anterior costophrenic angle where the lung is displaced superiorly. Note that there is no discernable difference in density when the lung is displaced posteriorly because the amount of lung tissue has not altered, only the air within the lung has been replaced by air outside the lung.

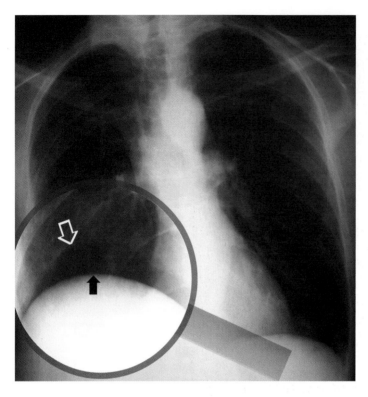

Figure 11.24. AP semi-erect CXR of an adult with a pneumothorax.

Due to the positioning of the patient there is no obvious lung edge with the free air situated in the anterior part of the hemithorax. The only clue is the very sharp right hemi-diaphragmatic silhouette (black arrow) and the just discernable inferior lung edge (open white arrow).

Similarly, anterior or posterior loculated pneumothoraces, which can occur following trauma or intervention, may be difficult to identify (*Fig. 11.25*).

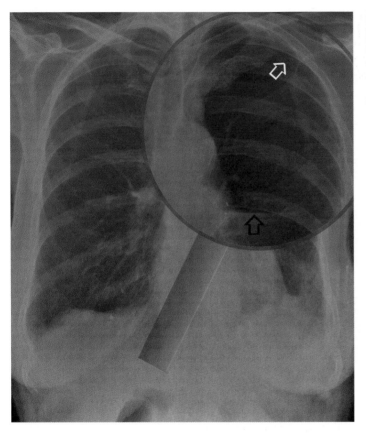

Figure 11.25. Frontal CXR of an adult with a loculated pneumothorax.

In this case the presence of the pneumothorax is evident from the lateral lung edge (open white arrow), but the presence of a small air–fluid level (open black arrow) indicates that there is also a locule of free air and fluid.

If an anterior pneumothorax is suspected (*Fig. 11.26*), a lateral horizontal CXR with the patient supine may identify the lung edge hidden on the frontal view; similarly, a lateral decubitus view may reveal the same. If the patient is well enough, a volume CT scan is the most accurate way to tease out difficult pneumothoraces, giving a clearer idea of their site, extent, nature and feasibility for drainage.

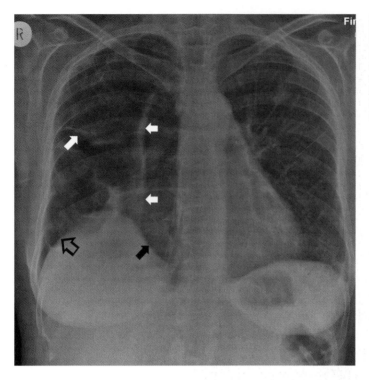

Figure 11.26. Frontal CXR of an adult with a complex loculated anterior pneumothorax.

Note the difference in clarity of the hemi-diaphragmatic silhouette resulting from free air in the pneumothorax (black arrow) compared to that formed by adjacent aerated lung (open black arrow). Other lung edges are also seen (white arrows).

11.3 Pleural thickening

It is difficult on CXR to distinguish basal pleural thickening from effusions when the only sign is blunting of the costophrenic angle. Furthermore, pleural thickening of the anterior and posterior pleura, orientated *en face* to the incident X-rays, may not be seen at all, or at best as a subtle increase in density. Lateral pleural thickening is in a better orientation to be identified on CXR. If the pleural thickening is calcified it becomes more evident (*Fig. 11.27*); the main causes are asbestos exposure, previous empyema (particularly TB) and previous haemothorax (*Fig. 11.28*; see also *Fig. 6.17*).

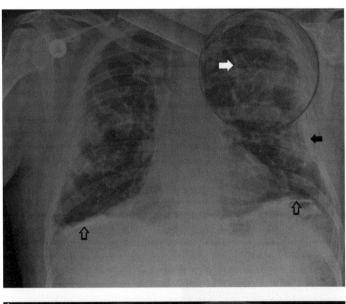

(a)

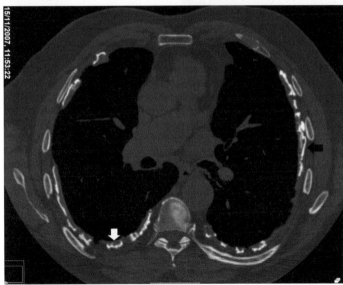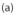

(b)

Figure 11.27. Frontal CXR (a) and axial CT image (b) of an adult male previously exposed to asbestos dust.

Note the bilateral calcified pleural plaques appearing denser over the hemi-diaphragms (open black arrows) and laterally (black arrows) where they are in line with the incident X-rays better than those seen *en face* (white arrows).

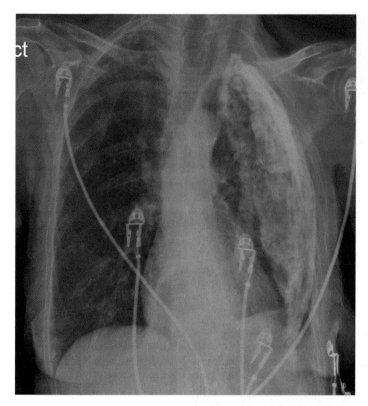

Figure 11.28. Frontal CXR demonstrating dense unilateral pleural calcification.

In this case the pleural calcification resulted from previous TB empyema.

The pleural surface is curved and as such is only in line with the incident X-rays of a CXR at particular margins: the mediastinal silhouette, the hemi-diaphragmatic silhouette and the lateral chest wall. Pleural thickening and calcification at these sites are seen end on and readily appreciated. It is the pleural thickening elsewhere that is often hidden and, when calcified, causes subtle areas of increased density that mimic lung parenchymal lesions (*Figs 11.29* and *11.30*).

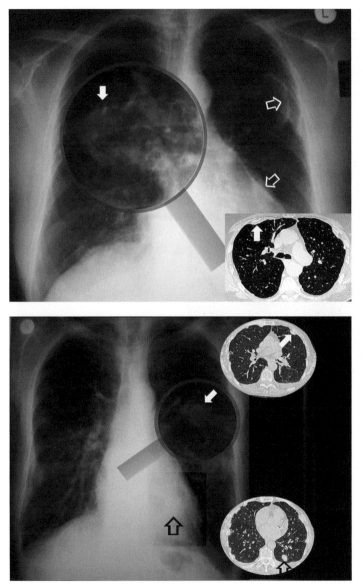

Figure 11.29. Frontal CXR and inset axial HRCT image of an adult with extensive calcified pleural plaques secondary to asbestos exposure.

Where these plaques are imaged side-on they can readily be identified (open white arrow), but when *en face* they may mimic pulmonary nodules (white arrow), and axial imaging may be the only way to clarify the appearances.

Figure 11.30. Frontal CXR and inset CT images of an adult with multiple calcified pleural plaques.

En face the plaques can mimic a nodule (white arrow); in this case there is also a primary lung malignancy 'hidden' behind the heart (open black arrow).

11.4 Pleural malignancy

The following features of pleural thickening suggest malignant rather than benign aetiology: thickness greater than 1 cm, nodular or undulating surface, involvement of the mediastinal pleura, encasement of the lung, and evidence of chest wall invasion; all of these are potentially visible on a CXR, depending on the size of the tumour.

The main malignant tumours of the pleura are mesothelioma (a sequel of asbestos exposure; see *Fig. 11.31*) and metastatic disease (usually adenocarcinoma; see *Figs 11.32* and *11.33*); in addition, although rare, pleural extension of a thymic malignancy may occur. Distinguishing these can be difficult, but features favouring mesothelioma are the presence of calcified plaques, indicating a previous exposure to asbestos, and contraction of the affected hemithorax, often in excess of the degree of thickening. One of the earliest signs of mesothelioma is a unilateral pleural effusion (*Fig. 11.34*), for which there is a wide differential, but also associated with loss of volume in the affected hemithorax.

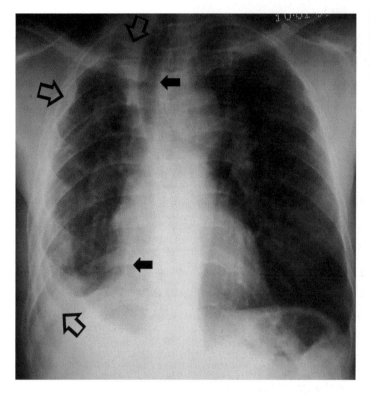

Figure 11.31. Frontal CXR of an adult with mesothelioma.

Note the encasing pleural thickening (open black arrows) and loss of volume in the affected hemithorax, causing mediastinal shift (black arrows).

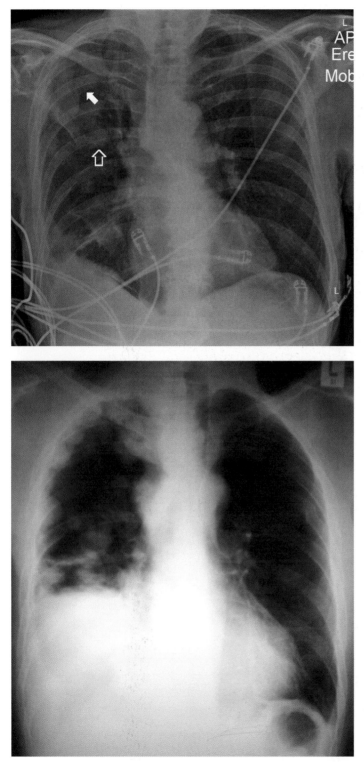

Figure 11.32. AP CXR of an adult with adenocarcinoma metastases to the pleura.

Note the nodular opacity with only the medial margin well defined (open white arrow), and the pleural nodule seen *en face* causing a rounded opacity (white arrow).

Figure 11.33. Frontal CXR of an adult with adenocarcinoma metastases to the right pleura.

Note the nodularity and encasement of the lung. This demonstrates how asymmetrical pleural metastases can be and they can therefore mimic mesothelioma; if this were mesothelioma one would expect some associated volume loss in the right hemithorax.

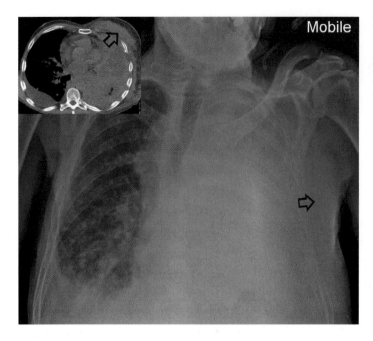

Figure 11.34. Frontal CXR with an axial CT image inset of an adult male patient with extensive mesothelioma.

The tumour occupies the entire left hemithorax and soft tissue extension into the chest wall is evident (open black arrow). There are multiple metastatic nodules on the right and a right-sided pleural effusion.

11.5 Benign pleural tumours

Benign pleural tumours are not common, they can grow to be very large before detection (*Fig. 11.35*) and, when pedunculated in nature, may appear to arise from the lung parenchyma as they will form an acute angle with the chest wall. Most are fibrous stromal tumours and can be difficult to excise completely with a high recurrence rate.

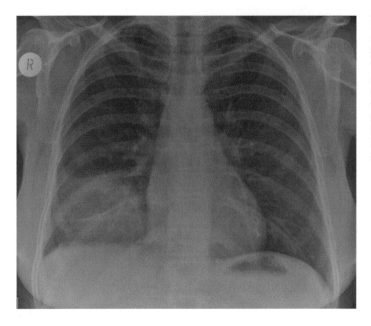

Figure 11.35. Frontal CXR of an adult with a large pleural fibroma arising posteriorly in the right lower zone.

This is actually a recurrence of already resected disease; these tumours are difficult to completely excise. The posterior site can be ascertained from the preservation of the right hemidiaphragmatic silhouette; the presence of visible lung vasculature implies, given its size, that this is a peripheral lesion, but its pleural origin cannot be confirmed on this CXR.

12 Left heart failure

Left heart failure describes the inability of the heart to pump all the blood that arrives from the pulmonary circulation into the aorta, causing a build-up of pressure in the pulmonary venous system. The result is accumulation of extra-vascular fluid in the interstitium of the lung. If the amount of fluid or pressure in the interstitium becomes too great the fluid will 'leak' into the air spaces, interlobular septa and the pleural space. 'Leak' is a convenient descriptive term, but in actuality the accumulation of fluid in these spaces is due to an imbalance in a production / absorption equilibrium. The most common cardiac changes associated with prolonged left heart failure are due to persistent raised pressure, resulting in enlargement of the left atrium and left ventricle (see *Section 13.2*).

The first sign of this process on a CXR is upper lobe blood diversion and lower lobe vasoconstriction (*Fig. 12.1*); the vessels being altered are the pulmonary veins. As fluid accumulates in the interstitium the venules are compressed, and this is more marked in the dependent lower zones of the chest, assuming the patient is erect in posture. The increased vascular resistance results in the diversion of blood preferentially into the upper lobes, causing an increase in calibre of the upper lobe pulmonary veins and reduction in calibre of the lower lobe pulmonary veins. Note that prominent upper lobe veins are not enough for this sign, there must be upper lobe blood diversion and lower lobe vasoconstriction.

The order in which the signs of heart failure manifest are not rigidly defined, but interstitial thickening causing reticulation on the CXR (*Fig. 12.2*) usually precedes air space filling that causes ground glass opacification (*Fig. 12.3*) and, subsequently, consolidation termed pulmonary oedema (*Fig. 12.4*). This sequence of events typically occurs in a peri-hilar distribution, sparing the lower zones and periphery in the first instance. This has given rise to the descriptive term 'bat's wing opacity'.

Fluid accumulates in the interlobular septa, giving rise to septal lines (see *Fig. 4.24*), and in the pleural space, resulting in pleural effusions (see *Fig. 11.2*) which, on CXR, may appear unilateral. In some instances the dependent fluid accumulation at the costophrenic angles is imaged while still within the substance of the lung. This gives rise to the rather inappropriately named lamellar effusions which present as a peripheral band of density in the lower zones (*Fig. 12.5*).

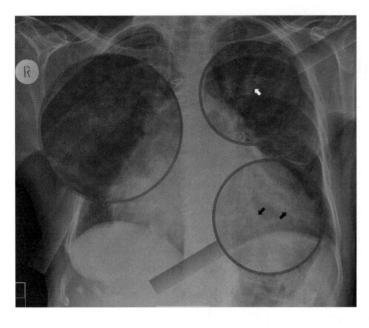

Figure 12.1. AP CXR of a patient in early left heart failure.

Note the dilated upper lobe veins (white arrows) and constricted lower lobe veins (black arrows). In addition, the vascular markings in the magnified area on the right are less distinct due to interstitial oedema.

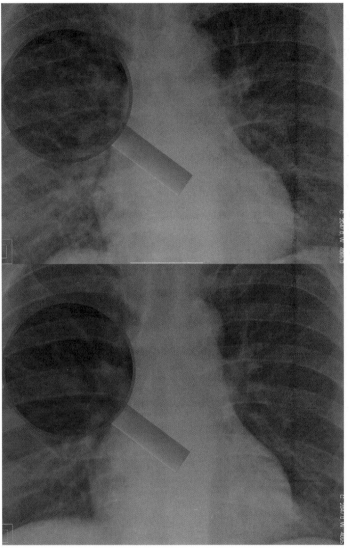

Figure 12.2. Representative images from two CXRs of the same patient taken 2 days apart.

The upper image demonstrates interstitial pulmonary oedema with reticular shadowing causing the vascular markings to become indistinct. Compare the appearances with the earlier lower image taken before the patient went into left heart failure. There is no consolidation in the upper image; the vessels are not completely obscured.

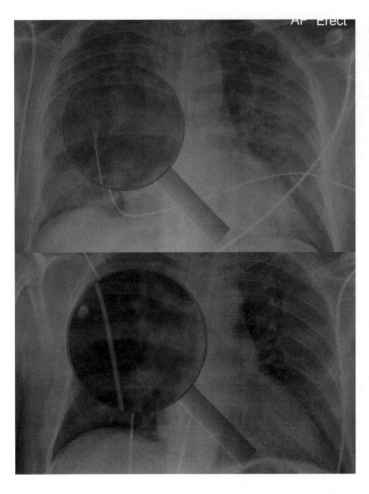

Figure 12.3. Representative images from two CXRs of the same patient taken 4 days apart.

On the upper later image there is ground glass opacity due to left heart failure obscuring the vessels, but not causing air-bronchograms. For comparison, the bottom image shows the earlier more normal CXR.

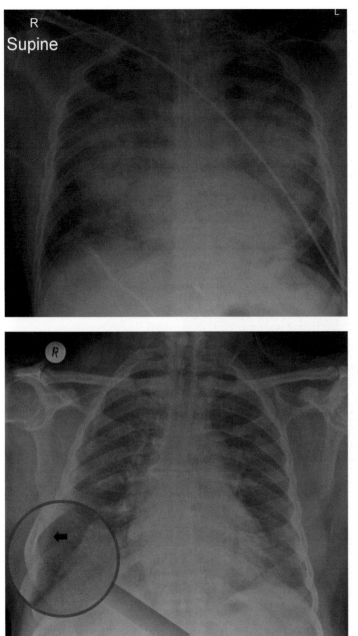

Figure 12.4. A supine CXR on an adult in left heart failure.

Note the bilateral peri-hilar consolidation: 'bat's wing opacity'. In addition to the heart failure, careful scrutiny reveals the tip of the endo-tracheal tube is at the carina and therefore too low.

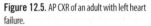

Figure 12.5. AP CXR of an adult with left heart failure.

The peripheral linear opacification (black arrow) corresponds to a lamellar pleural effusion.

13 The heart and great vessels

Recognition of cardiac and great vessel abnormalities on a CXR depends upon appreciating changes in the mediastinal silhouette and / or observing the effect of the abnormality on the lung vasculature.

The main pathology associated with the heart is enlargement or hypertrophy. Cardiac size is determined by measuring the maximum horizontal contour on a PA CXR (*Fig. 13.1*); this measurement should not be diagonal! The upper limit of normal for a male is 16 cm and for a female is 15 cm. Note that this measurement does not consider the trans-thoracic diameter. The calculation of a cardio–thoracic ratio (CTR) should be reserved for serial measurements of cardiac size to determine whether there is any change in size, rather than as an absolute measure. Conventional teaching suggests that a CTR of >50% indicates cardiac enlargement, but in some adult patients the trans-thoracic diameter is less than 28 cm, which would allow them a maximum cardiac diameter of only 14 cm.

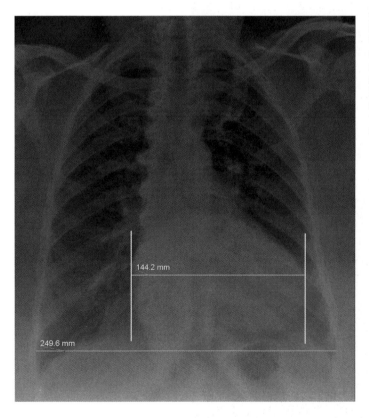

144.2 mm

249.6 mm

Figure 13.1. Calculating cardiac size.

The heart size, in this case 14.4 cm, is the horizontal distance between the two vertical lines marking the edges of the heart borders. The trans-thoracic diameter, 25 cm in this case, is the maximum horizontal distance between the inner margin of opposite ribs. Note that the CTR in this case is 14.5 / 25, i.e. >50%, but the heart size is actually normal.

13.1 Valve replacements

There are numerous different makes of prosthetic valve that are variably visible on CXR. The prosthetic valve itself may be seen or alternatively the supporting structure for a tissue valve. Usually the projection of the valve on the CXR is sufficient to localise it (*Fig. 13.2*).

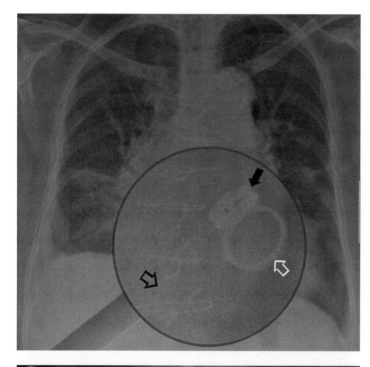

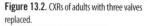

Figure 13.2. CXRs of adults with three valves replaced.

(a) Frontal CXR of an adult with three valves replaced: the mitral (open white arrow), aortic (black arrow) and tricuspid (open black arrow) valves. Note that the mitral and tricuspid valves are larger than the aortic valve and, compared to the other two, the aortic valve is seen more side-on. The aortic valve is sited in the middle of the heart, the mitral lower to the left, and the tricuspid the lowest and to the right; if present the pulmonary valve would be seen side-on like the aortic valve to its right and orientated to point up and left.
(b) Frontal CXR with the same three valves replaced as in (a): the aortic (black arrow), mitral (open white arrow) and tricuspid (open black arrow) valves. Note that the relative positions are the same as in (a), but the aortic prosthetic valve is of a different type.

(a)

(b)

13.2 Cardiac enlargement

Typically associated with heart failure secondary to mitral valve disease, cardiomegaly is readily appreciated on CXR, but the functional significance can only be assumed by associated CXR signs of heart failure. The apex of the heart is displaced laterally and slightly inferiorly and, in the context of mitral valve disease, there may be signs of left atrial enlargement: dilated left atrial appendage, double heart border and splayed carina (*Fig. 13.3*).

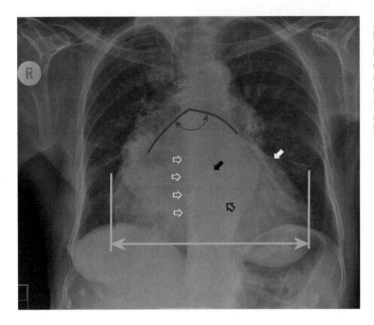

Figure 13.3. Frontal CXR on an adult female.

Note the sternotomy wires indicating previous cardiac surgery (open white arrows), aortic (black arrow) and mitral (open black arrow) valve replacements, and a dilated left atrial appendage (white arrow) which, along with the widened carinal angle, indicate left atrial enlargement. Again note the technique for measuring cardiac size.

Left and right ventricular hypertrophy cause a less marked cardiac enlargement and tend to elevate the cardiac apex (*Fig. 13.4*). Right atrial enlargement is unusual and causes increased convexity to the right heart silhouette.

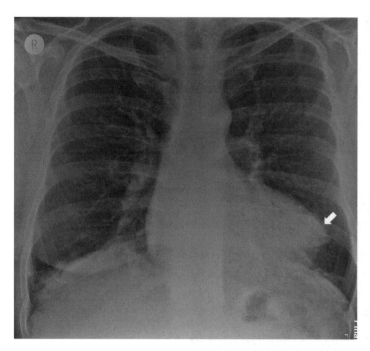

Figure 13.4. Frontal CXR of an adult with right ventricular hypertrophy secondary to primary pulmonary hypertension.

Note the elevation of the apex of the heart (white arrow) giving rise to a 'boot shaped' appearance.

13.3 Ventricular aneurysm

The myocardium following an infarct becomes replaced by fibrous tissue that may calcify (*Fig. 13.5*) or, under continuous pressure, allow the bulging of the left ventricular wall forming an aneurysm (*Fig. 13.6*). As a result, the cardiac contour is altered and the heart size enlarged. Differentiation from dilated cardiomegaly may be difficult but, as the aneurysmal wall is static, the underlying blood stasis promotes thrombus formation. Curvilinear calcification of the mural thrombus may be seen on CXR and reveals the true cause of the cardiac enlargement.

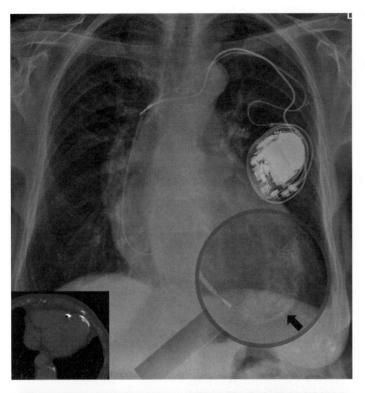

Figure 13.5. Frontal CXR and inset CT image of an adult after an infarct.

Note the calcification in the region of the cardiac apex (black arrow) confirmed to represent calcified myocardium in the CT image.

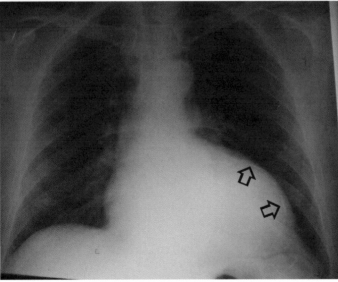

Figure 13.6. Frontal CXR of an adult with a left ventricular aneurysm.

Note the more convex left heart border and the curvilinear calcification (open black arrows) inside the myocardium, unlike pericardial calcification which would be on the surface.

13.4 Pericardial disease

A pericardial effusion (*Fig. 13.7*) can cause a global enlargement of the cardiac silhouette. The convexity of the right heart border and filling out of the border defined by the left atrial appendage, gives an overall *globular* appearance. The diagnosis is readily confirmed at echocardiography, but comparison with previous CXRs is of great help in making the diagnosis radiologically (*Fig. 13.8*) and the development of the pericardial effusion can be quantified by the CTR.

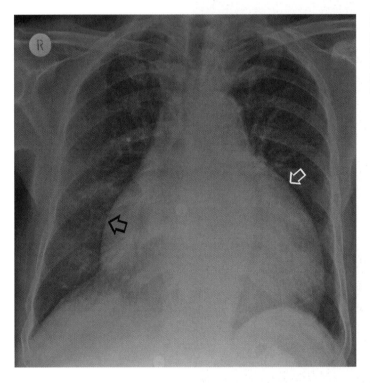

Figure 13.7. Frontal CXR of an adult with a large pericardial effusion.

Note the globular contour to the heart, primarily due to increased convexity of the right heart border (open black arrow) and the region of the left atrial appendage (open white arrow).

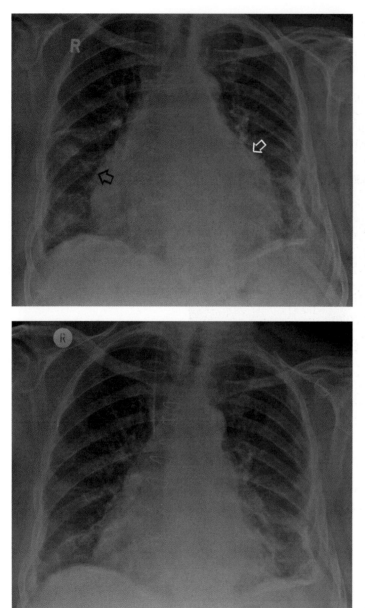

(a)

(b)

Figure 13.8. AP CXRs of an adult in the week following cardiac surgery.

(a) This demonstrates a large pericardial effusion, changing the heart shape to globular through the increased convexity of the cardiac margins, particularly in the region of the aortic outflow tract (open black arrow) and the left atrial appendage (open white arrow). This occurred 3 days after removal of epicardial pacing wires which caused a haemopericardium.

(b) CXR taken on the day the epicardial wires were removed. Note how the contour of the heart has changed as the pericardium filled with fluid.

Inflammation of the pericardium may heal with fibrosis causing cardiac constriction and this may be discernable on CXR if the fibrosis calcifies (*Fig. 13.9*).

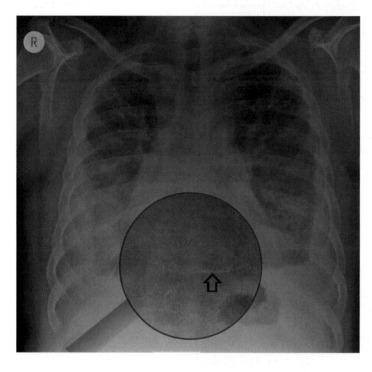

Figure 13.9. AP CXR on an adult.

Note in the magnified area the curvilinear lines due to pericardial calcification (open black arrow). Elsewhere on the CXR are signs of left heart failure with bilateral pleural effusions and peri-hilar interstitial pulmonary oedema.

13.5 Coarctation of the aorta

Coarctation of the aorta is a congenital narrowing of the thoracic aorta, usually at the isthmus where the aortic arch becomes the descending aorta (*Fig. 13.10*). As the anomaly is present at birth, the reduction in blood flow to the lower half of the body can be compensated for by recruiting the intercostals vessels as conduits from the unaffected upper body arterial circulation to the aorta distal to the coarctation. As the intercostal vessels enlarge to take on this increased flow, they erode the underside of the rib at the point where the flange of the rib begins, causing rib notching; the narrowing of the aorta and post-stenotic dilation may give a contour to the aortic knuckle, resembling a '3'. Coarctation usually presents in early adulthood when the collateral arterial supply to the lower body becomes insufficient. Even if the coarctation is corrected the rib notching will persist.

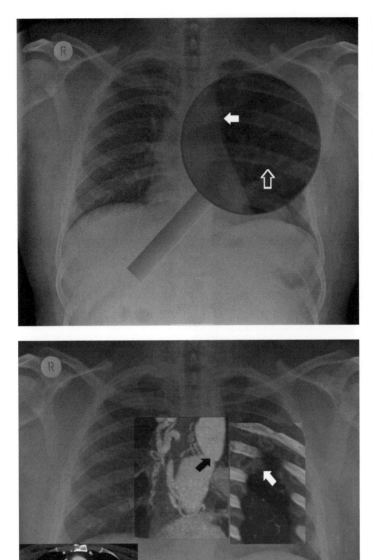

Figure 13.10. Coarctation of the aorta.

(a) Frontal CXR on an adult with aortic coarctation. Note the diminutive aortic knuckle (white arrow) and the rib notching (open white arrow).

(b) Same CXR with coronal reconstructions from a CT scan of the same patient at the same time, and an axial image at the level of the coarctation. Note the narrowing of the aorta (black arrow) and the dilated intercostal artery giving rise to the rib notching (white arrow). There are many of these dilated intercostal arteries contributing to the collateral blood supply to the aorta distal to the coarctation (open white arrow).

(a)

(b)

13.6 Aortic aneurysm

The course of the aorta is such that only one side of it is seen on a frontal CXR (*Fig. 13.11*), except when the descending aorta is very tortuous. As a result one must distinguish true aneurysmal dilatation from a tortuous normal calibre aorta (*Figs 13.12–13.14*). When the aneurysm causes a definable alteration in the aortic contour the task is relatively straightforward. Similarly, aneurysmal dilatation in the region of the arch and isthmus are difficult to mimic through unfolding, but a fusiform aneurysm of the ascending or descending aorta may prove to be a tougher proposition, and if a lateral view fails to help, a limited CT scan can be performed (just a few 5 mm slices through the region of concern).

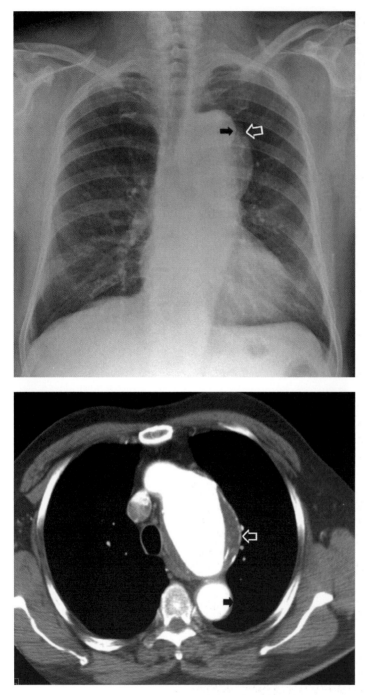

(a)

(b)

Figure 13.11. Frontal chest radiograph (a) and contrast-enhanced axial CT image (b) of an adult with an aneurysm of the aortic arch.

Note the two silhouettes, one corresponding to the normal descending aorta (black arrow) and the other generated by the aneurysm (white arrow).

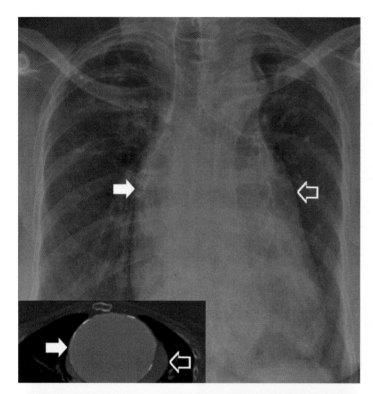

(a)

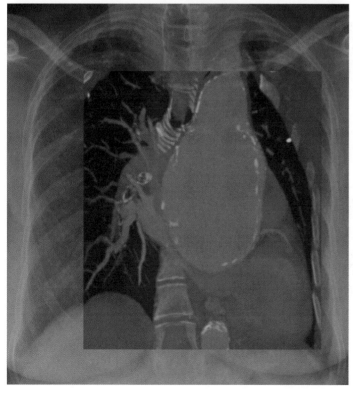

(b)

Figure 13.12. Adult with a large ascending aortic aneurysm.

(a) Frontal CXR with an axial image inset. Note that the right-sided margin seen on the CXR is formed by the aorta (white arrow), but on the left, even in an aneurysm of this size, the margin seen on a PA CXR is due to displacement of a normal mediastinal structure, in this case the atrial appendage.
(b) Same CXR with a coronal CT image superimposed.

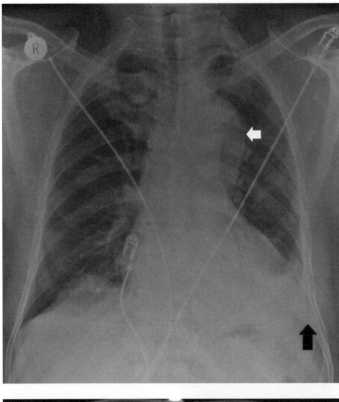

Figure 13.13. Frontal CXR (a) and contrast-enhanced axial CT image (b) of an adult patient with acute aortic dissection.

Note the aneurysmal aortic arch and the unilateral left pleural effusion indicating an acute event. Clinical history of central chest pain radiating to the back assisted in this diagnosis, and dissection was confirmed on CT imaging.

(a)

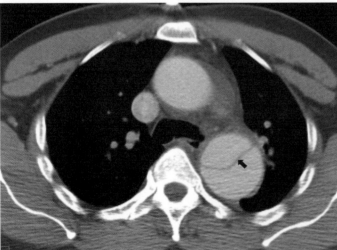

(b)

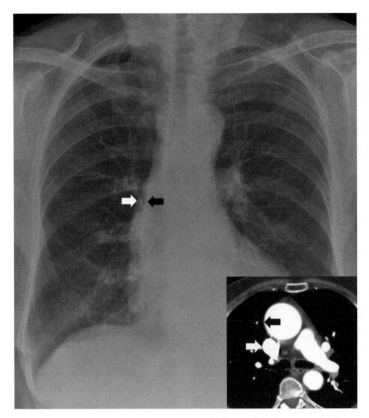

Figure 13.14. Frontal CXR of an adult with an axial CT section inset.

There is dilatation of the ascending aorta resulting in two visible contours, that of the aorta (black arrow) and that of the SVC (white arrow). The interface between aerated lung and a normal calibre ascending aorta is normally oblique to the incident X-rays and therefore not seen.

13.7 Atrial septal defect

Atrial septal defect is a congenital patent communication between the atria. As the left atrium is at a higher pressure than the right atrium, blood passes from left to right: a right to left shunt. As a result there is an increase in pulmonary arterial flow and pressure, and this may become apparent on CXR due to an increase in diameter and tortuosity of the proximal pulmonary arterial vessels; these may return to normal following repair of the defect (*Fig. 13.15*).

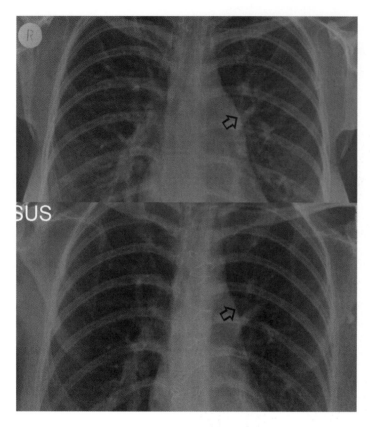

Figure 13.15. Two portions of CXRs taken from the same adult.

The upper image is before corrective surgery for an atrial septal defect and the lower image is following surgery. Note the change in the convexity of the pulmonary outflow tract (open black arrows) when dilated before, and normal calibre after, surgery. The peri-hilar vascularity, particularly in the mid zones, is reduced following surgery. Appearances in the upper pre-surgery image can be described as plethoric.

13.8 Pacemakers

There are an increasingly varied number of cardiac pacemakers and defibrillators both permanent and temporary. Below (*Figs 13.16–13.21*) are examples of the most common pacemakers and some of the positioning errors that may be detected on CXR.

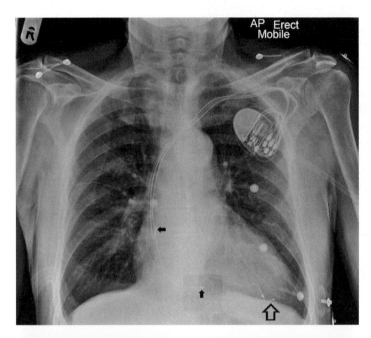

Figure 13.16. Frontal CXR of an adult with a three lead pacemaker.

There are the usual right atrial and right ventricular leads (black arrows), but also a lead in the coronary venous sinus that paces the left ventricle (open black arrow).

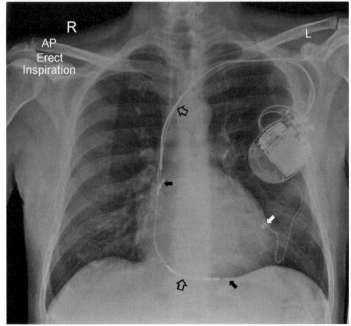

Figure 13.17. AP CXR of an adult with an intracardiac defibrillator with external left ventricular pacing.

The right atrial and right ventricular lead (black arrows) and the left ventricular lead (white arrow) are marked. The defibrillator leads can be identified by the thickened sections (open black arrows).

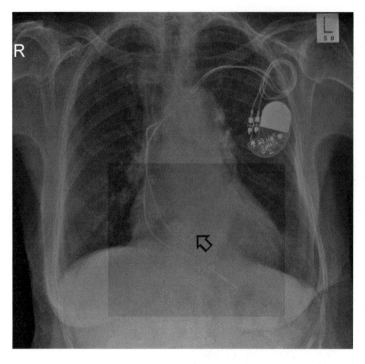

Figure 13.18. Frontal CXR of an adult with a dual chamber permanent pacemaker.

Note that the right atrial lead (open black arrow) is incorrectly placed in the right ventricle.

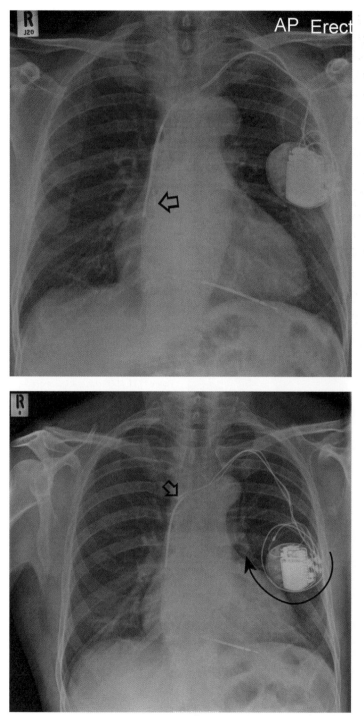

(a)

(b)

Figure 13.19. Frontal CXRs of an adult with a dual chamber permanent pacemaker.

(a) Note the position of the right atrial lead (open black arrow).
(b) Frontal CXR of the same patient. The pacemaker has been rotated by the patient repetitively fiddling with it and, as a result, the right atrial lead has become displaced (open black arrow).

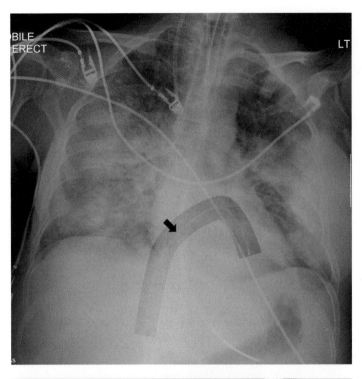

Figure 13.20. AP CXR of an adult with ARDS following a cardiac arrest.

Note the bilateral dependent dense consolidation. There is a temporary pacing wire *in situ*, inserted via the right femoral vein / IVC route (black arrow).

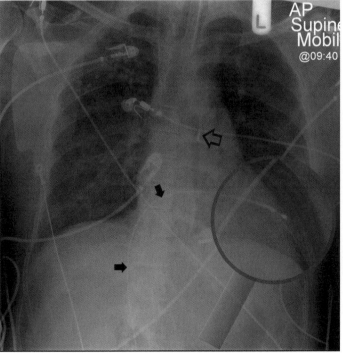

Figure 13.21. AP CXR of an adult following cardiac arrest.

A temporary pacing wire has been placed via the right femoral vein (black arrows). Note the tip of the wire (magnified area) extends to the pericardium and has therefore punctured the right ventricle. Temporary wires are often placed under duress with the patient unwell, so their positioning should be carefully scrutinised. Clues to this patient's clinical state are the presence of a balloon pump (open black arrow) and a defibrillator pad visible on the patient's chest.

14 Pulmonary embolic disease

The main value of a CXR in suspected acute pulmonary embolus (PE) is in identifying other possible causes for the PE, like symptoms such as pneumothorax, pneumonia, etc. In a PE the CXR is usually normal and, in the context of a normal CXR, a perfusion scan alone may be a suitable test for PE because the CXR can be taken to indicate normal ventilation. Vessels filled with thrombus / embolus cast the same shadow on a CXR as those filled with blood, and so a PE will only become apparent if the distal vessels empty of blood. However, there is no negative pressure from the left side of the heart to 'suck' this blood through the lungs so it becomes static and clots, leaving the vessel unchanged on a CXR (*Fig. 14.1*). In the presence of an abnormal CXR, a definitive diagnosis of PE from ventilation / perfusion (V/Q) scanning is unlikely and CT pulmonary angiography may be more useful. In the relatively rare case of pulmonary infarction, the matching of perfusion and ventilation defects with lung opacification may be found: a 'triple match'. Conventionally, V/Q scanning is aimed at identifying mismatches whereby an aerated area of lung has no blood supply.

CXR abnormalities associated with, but not specific to, a PE are pleural effusion, atelectasis and paucity of vascular markings. When infarcted, sub-segmental areas of the lung may cause wedge-shaped opacities on CXR which may cavitate (*Fig. 14.2*).

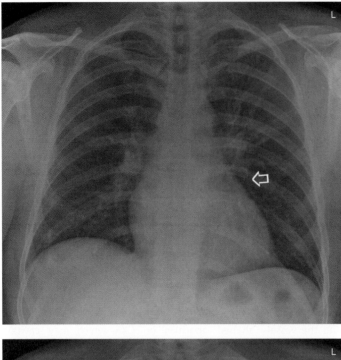

(a)

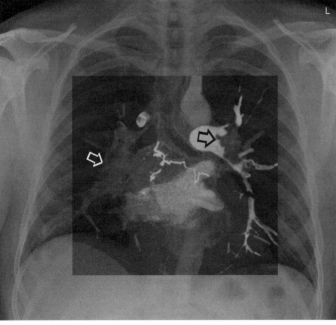

(b)

Figure 14.1. Adult with massive bilateral pulmonary emboli.

(a) Frontal CXR; the most striking aspect is how normal the CXR appears. With hindsight there may be a cut-off to the left basal pulmonary artery (open white arrow), but the bulk of the embolus is actually on the right basal pulmonary arteries. (b) Same CXR with a coronal reconstruction from the subsequent CT scan. This demonstrates the position of the embolus in the LLL artery (open black arrow), but note the more dramatic lack of contrast on the right (open white arrow). As the left-sided embolus is causing incomplete obstruction, the blood flow diminishes rather than ceases, allowing the vessel to partially empty such that the calibre change is just discernable on the CXR. On the right the vessels have thrombosed and they retain their original calibre.

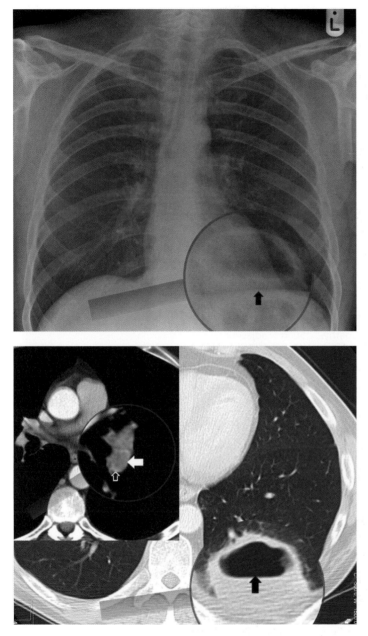

(a)

(b)

Figure 14.2. Patient with a cavitating lesion in the left lower lobe.

(a) Frontal CXR; note the normal left hemi-diaphragmatic silhouette (black arrow) indicating that this lesion is in the lung and probably not related to the diaphragm.

(b) Axial CT images from the same case demonstrating the posteriorly placed LLL cavity. Note the air–fluid level (black arrow), increasing the suspicion that there is a secondary infection. The inset image is from a superior slice from the same CT scan and demonstrates an embolus (white arrow) in the LLL artery, outlined by intravenous contrast (open white arrow).

15 The mediastinum

The margins of the mediastinum adjacent to aerated lung are readily seen, but the only natural contrast between the mediastinal structures themselves is provided by mediastinal fat, and these interfaces are not readily seen on CXR. As a result, mediastinal pathology may be very difficult to identify on CXR unless it affects the mediastinal silhouette and, as a result, is readily underestimated.

If there is evidence of extra soft tissue in the mediastinum, a clue as to the nature of that tissue may be derived from its location. Tumours of the mediastinum anterior to the heart are conveniently summarised as the 'terrible Ts'; Thyroid, Teratoma, Thymoma, Terrible lymphadenopathy. Such pathology is readily hidden between the heart and sternum on a frontal CXR, but will eventually affect the mediastinal silhouette, characteristically obscuring the heart border but sparing the hilar point. On a lateral film, the abnormal anterior mediastinal soft tissue is more readily seen filling the normally 'clear' triangle behind the sternum (*Fig. 15.1*).

Elsewhere in the mediastinum, the differentials become longer but identifying a posterior / paraspinal mass, preserving both the cardiac silhouette and the hilar point, is worthwhile because it should lead to careful scrutiny of the adjacent spine.

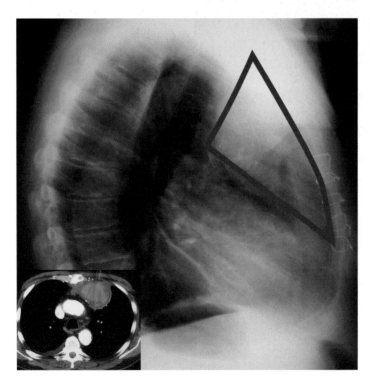

Figure 15.1. Lateral CXR and inset CT image of an adult with an anterior mediastinal mass.

Note the 'filling in' of the retro-sternal triangle.

15.1 The 'hidden' areas of the mediastinum

Identifying a mass bulging from the mediastinal contour is relatively straightforward, leaving only the antero–posterior position to be elucidated. The challenge is in identifying abnormal soft tissue that is not so readily appreciated. In the anatomy section (*Chapter 2*) the various mediastinal lines were described and this is where we put that knowledge to use.

The azygo–oesophageal line should be seen overlying the spine inferior to the carina. It is formed by the combination of aerated lung next to the azygous and / or the oesophagus in line with the incident X-rays. If there is abnormal soft tissue in the sub-carinal region this will alter the contour of the azygo–oesophageal line, causing it either to bulge or changing the orientation of the soft tissue / aerated lung interface such that the line is no longer visible. Note that the azygo–oesophageal line may not be seen at all but this is very unlikely to be due to pathology:

- the loss of the azygo–oesophageal line superiorly suggests sub-carinal lymphadenopathy (*Figs15.2* and *15.3*)
- loss of the line inferiorly suggests a hiatus hernia (*Figs 15.4* and *15.5*) or lower oesophageal dilatation / mass

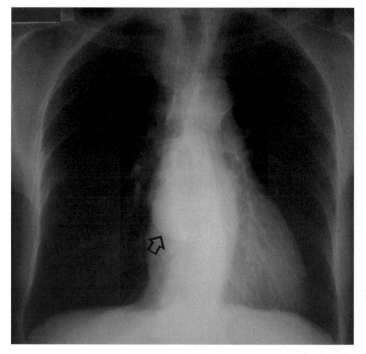

Figure 15.2. Frontal CXR of an adult.

Note the bulge to the azygo–oesophageal line (open black arrow) caused by sub-carinal adenopathy.

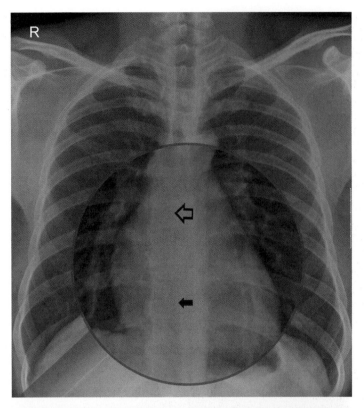

Figure 15.3. Frontal CXR of an adult with mediastinal lymphadenopathy.

The azygo–oesophageal line is visible (black arrow) but is then lost (open black arrow) due to sub-carinal adenopathy.

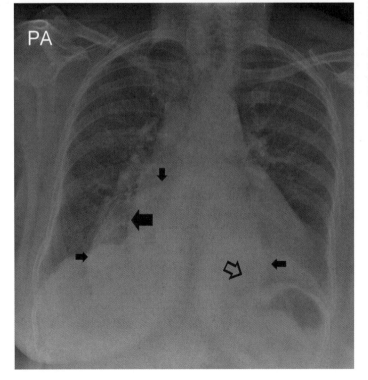

Figure 15.4. Frontal CXR of an adult with a large hiatus hernia.

The margins of the hernia are marked (small black arrows). Note that the 'top' is not seen as the oesophagus extends up from there. Note also the preservation of the right heart border (large black arrow) and the descending aortic (open black arrow) silhouettes.

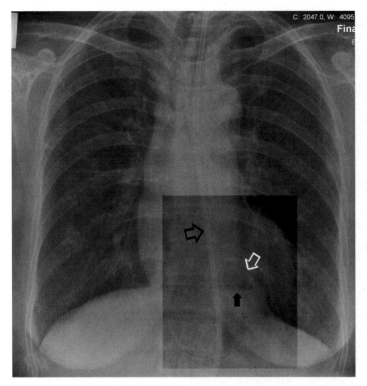

Figure 15.5. Frontal CXR of an adult with a small sliding hiatus hernia (open white arrow).

The naso-gastric tube reveals the course of the oesophagus (open black arrow) and the hernia contains an air–fluid level (black arrow). The absence of any inferior margin favours a sub-diaphragmatic origin, but a cavitating lesion abutting the diaphragm could have the same appearances; a limited CT scan through the area may be necessary to confirm the findings.

The right para-tracheal stripe (*Fig. 15.6*), formed by the combination of aerated lung adjacent to the right wall of the trachea, which itself is demarcated medially by the air in the trachea, is normally a maximum of 5 mm in thickness. Para-tracheal adenopathy will widen this stripe and can be readily identified on CXR (*Fig. 15.7*). Note that the azygous vein, as it courses anteriorly over the right main bronchus to drain into the SVC, forms the inferior margin of this stripe at the azygous knob where the stripe is inevitably greater than 5 mm in thickness. On a CXR the area adjacent to the right para-tracheal stripe is of increased density due to the SVC shadow. The SVC lies anterior to the trachea and so does not affect the stripe, but caution must be taken to avoid over-calling para-tracheal adenopathy due to the SVC shadow; the clue is in identifying the lateral margin of the stripe to determine its thickness. There is usually no left para-tracheal stripe to see, but lucency to the left of the trachea may indicate a dilated oesophagus or pneumomediastinum (see *Fig. 11.23a*).

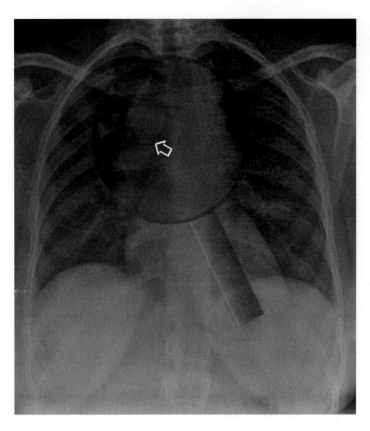

Figure 15.6. Frontal CXR of an adult with markedly enlarged right para-tracheal lymph nodes.

The medial margin of the tracheal wall is marked (open white arrow).

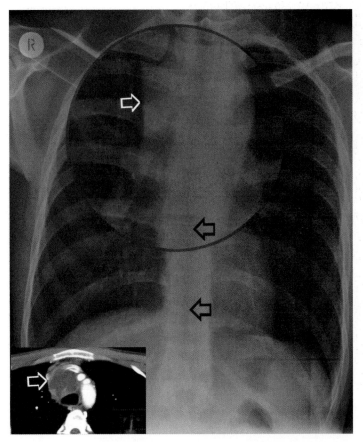

Figure 15.7. Frontal CXR and inset axial CT image of a patient with TB.

Note the large para-tracheal lymph node with central necrosis and peripheral enhancement (open white arrows) and, in comparison to *Figure 15.3*, the azygo–oesophageal line is easily seen (open black arrows).

The aorto–pulmonary (A–P) window describes the pocket of mediastinal tissue that lies lateral to the pulmonary outflow tract and the left main pulmonary artery, and infero-lateral to the aortic arch. It contains mainly fat and therefore normally appears as a concavity on the CXR, inferior to the aortic arch as described earlier. The main potentially pathological tissue in the A–P window is lymph nodes, and enlargement of these nodes may cause a filling-in or even a bulging of the A–P window (see *Fig. 4.39*). One significant feature of A–P window pathology is the possible involvement of the left recurrent laryngeal nerve that supplies the left vocal cord, thereby causing a hoarse voice. Developmentally this nerve is dragged into the thorax because it becomes tangled around the ductus arteriosus, bridging the aorta and the left main bronchus. No such 'trap' exists on the right side, so the right recurrent laryngeal nerve goes no lower than the root of the neck.

Bulging of the para-spinal lines indicates the presence of abnormal para-spinal soft tissue, and should prompt careful scrutiny of the adjacent vertebral bodies as a possible source of the pathology that may be evident on CXR, but axial imaging is usually required to delineate the cause (*Fig 15.8*). Just anterior to the para-spinal line is the lateral demarcation of the descending aorta; a large para-spinal mass may obscure this margin (*Fig. 15.9*).

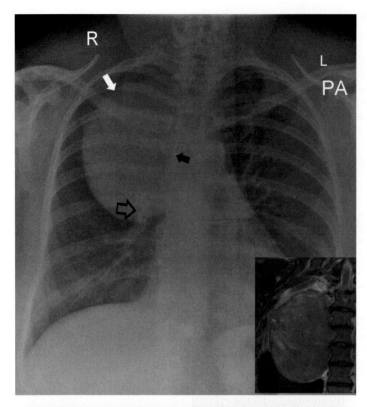

Figure 15.8. Frontal CXR of an adult with a large para-spinal mass and an inset coronal MRI image.

The posterior location of this mass is evident by the preservation of the para-tracheal stripe (black arrow) and the hilar vessels (open black arrow), the clarity of the lateral margin (white arrow), and extension above the projection of the clavicle, which marks the superior limit of the anterior half of the lung.

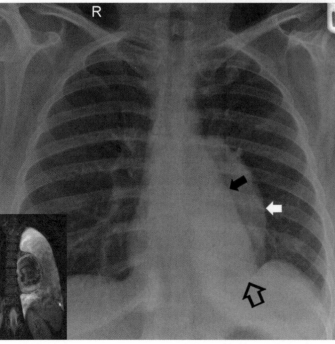

Figure 15.9. Frontal CXR and inset coronal MRI image of an adult with a large left-sided neurofibroma (black arrow).

The left heart border (black arrow) and left hemi-diaphragmatic silhouette (open black arrow) are seen but the descending aorta silhouette is obscured. The MRI demonstrates the mass that gives rise to the second silhouette (white arrow); because the patient is lying flat in the MRI scanner a small pleural effusion becomes visible on this image.

The anterior junctional line is too inconsistent for its absence to be taken as indicating pathology; a shame as it would be the ideal indicator of abnormal anterior mediastinal soft tissue that is not extensive enough to affect the mediastinal contours. In the presence of apparent mediastinal widening, the preservation of this junctional line would make the anterior mediastinum an unlikely site for the pathology.

The posterior junctional line may serve the same purpose as the anterior junctional line, only applied to the posterior mediastinum.

15.2 The hila

The anatomy of the hilar point is described in the anatomy section (see *Chapter 2*). Loss of the hilar point due to soft tissue density is usually the result of lymphadenopathy (*Fig. 15.10*), but could equally be due to a lung nodule or mass (*Fig. 15.11*). In addition to changes to the hilar point, there may be a discernable increase in the density of the hilum (*Fig. 15.12*). This is a harder sign to identify with confidence, as the only comparison is with the contra-lateral hilum and the orientation of the CXR may have a significant impact on the relative density of the hila.

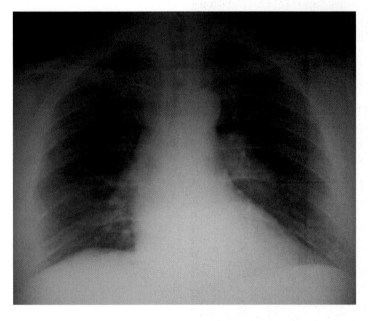

Figure 15.10. Frontal CXR of an adult with left hilar adenopathy.

Note the lobular contour to the hilum, but any increase in density is difficult to ascertain as the right hilum is obscured by an ecstatic ascending aorta.

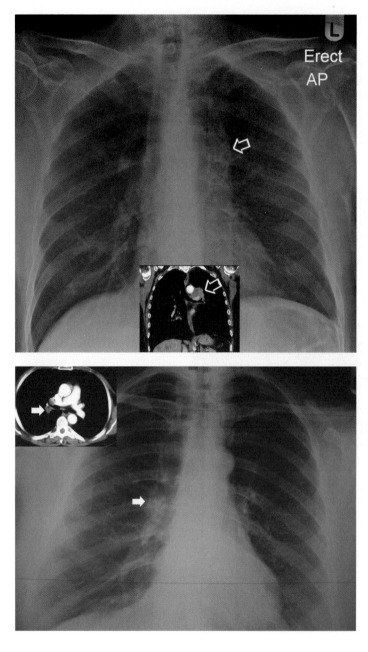

Figure 15.11. Frontal CXR of an adult with proximal primary lung cancer.

The cancer occupies the hilum and aorto–pulmonary window (open white arrow).

Figure 15.12. A–P CXR and inset CT image of an adult with hilar adenopathy (white arrow).

The amount of adenopathy is insufficient to alter the hilar contour, but there is a subtle increase in hilar density. The hilum is an area that even experienced radiologists interpret inaccurately.

15.3 Stents

The main structures in the mediastinum that may be stented to retain patency are the aorta, SVC (*Fig. 15.13*), innominate vein (*Fig. 15.14*), oesophagus (*Fig. 15.15*), and the trachea and main bronchi (*Fig. 15.16*). Stents are readily identified as tubular structures usually comprising a fine metallic meshwork; some oesophageal stents are non-metallic. They are deployed when there is extrinsic, and sometimes intrinsic, narrowing of a vital structure. Determining what has been stented relies on identifying the stent position in relation to the mediastinal anatomy.

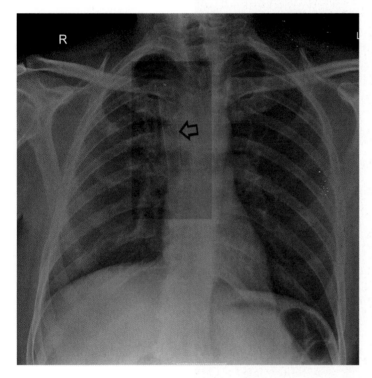

Figure 15.13. Frontal CXR of an adult with a right hilar lung cancer and mediastinal adenopathy that was compressing the SVC.

Note the metallic meshwork of the SVC stent in the highlighted region.

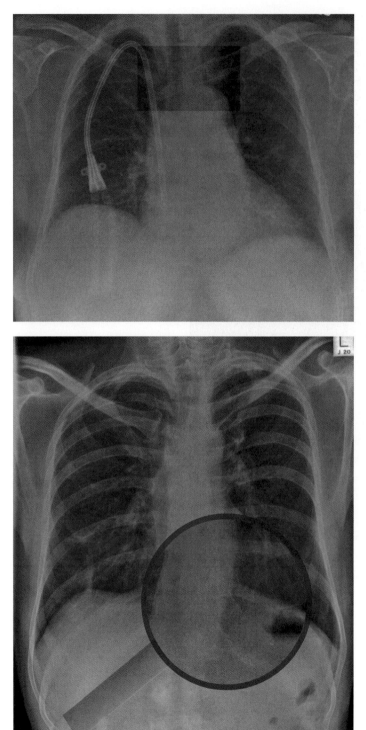

Figure 15.14. Frontal CXR of an adult with a vascular catheter *in situ* and a stent in the innominate vein.

Figure 15.15. Frontal CXR of an adult with oesophageal carcinoma.

Symptomatic relief has been achieved by the insertion of a lower oesophageal stent.

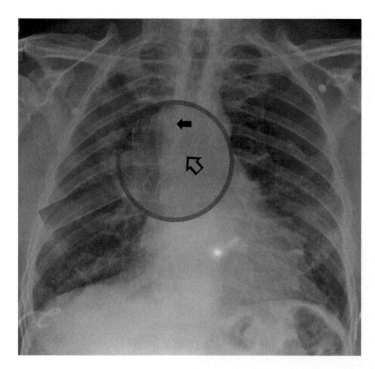

Figure 15.16. Frontal CXR of a patient with NSCLC.
Stents have been deployed in both the SVC (black arrow) and right main bronchus (open black arrow).

16 The ITU chest X-ray

The primary purpose of the ITU CXR is to confirm the position of the various intravenous lines, endo-tracheal tubes, naso-gastric tubes and other drainage tubes. The following imaging (*Figs 16.1–16.5*) demonstrates the type of tubes and lines that may be seen on an ITU CXR and indicates, where relevant, the ideal positioning.

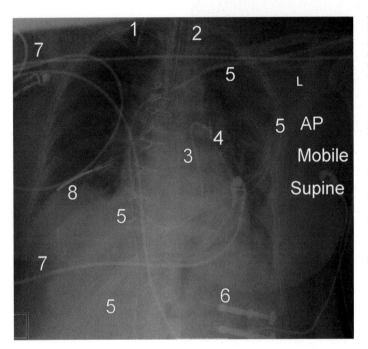

Figure 16.1. AP supine CXR of an adult patient on an ITU following a sternotomy.

Can you identify the various tubes and lines? Are they correctly placed?
The answers are as follows:
1. right internal jugular line; the tip is a little high but OK
2. endotracheal tube
3. Swaan–Gantz catheter; the tip rests in the pulmonary outflow tract, or main pulmonary artery as here
4. intra-aortic balloon pump; the radio-opaque tip should be as high as possible within the descending aorta but not into the arch; note the long inflated balloon below the tip
5. chest drains; these were put in at surgery, so although they are draining the pleural space they enter the thorax in the mid line
6. epicardial pacing; these are the contacts outside the patient for the epicardial pacing wires which themselves are very fine and difficult to see
7. ECG leads on the surface of the patient terminating with a clip attached to an ECG tab (not visible)
8. naso-gastric tube; note the long radio-opaque tip (unfortunately not all naso-gastric tube makes are this obvious on CXR); this naso-gastric tube is in the RLL and therefore incorrectly placed.

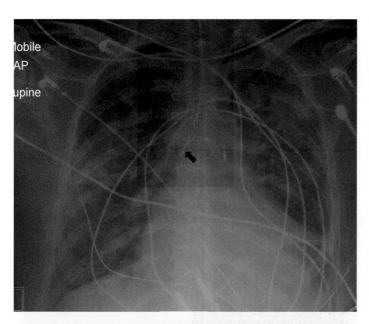

Figure 16.2. A semi-erect AP CXR of an adult being ventilated in ITU.

There are numerous lines seen, some inside and some on the surface of the patient. The key is to identify each and determine whether they are appropriately positioned. In this case the endo-tracheal tube is in the right main bronchus (black arrow) and needs to be withdrawn so that both lungs are ventilated.

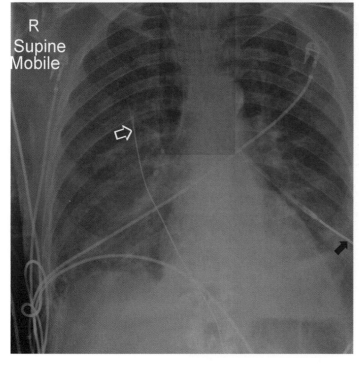

Figure 16.3. Supine CXR.

Note that the endo-tracheal tube and right internal jugular line are in satisfactory positions, and that the naso-gastric tube is misplaced down the left main bronchus. In addition, there is a surface wire with an indistinct end (open white arrow); this was the lead to an external pacing and defibrillator pad which itself is not radio-opaque.

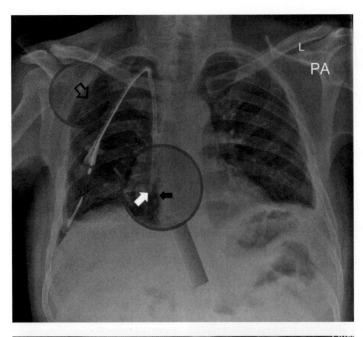

Figure 16.4. Frontal CXR of an adult.

Surprisingly this patient was well enough to have his CXR in the X-ray department. Attempted insertion of the central line has resulted in a pneumothorax (open black arrow); the line itself (white arrow) clearly lies lateral to the right atrium (black arrow) and therefore in the mediastinal tissues or pleural space.

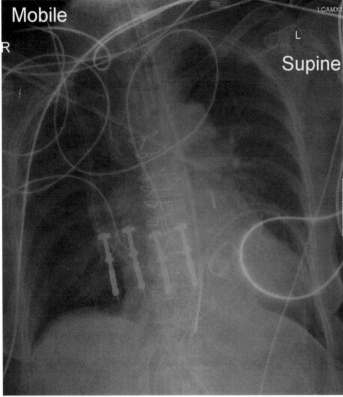

Figure 16.5. AP CXR of an adult ventilated on ITU.

Can you spot the incorrectly placed lines / tubes? The answer is as follows: the naso-gastric tube tip is in the lower oesophagus; the short linear radio-density overlying the descending aorta is the tip of a balloon catheter (not inflated on this image) and is far too low.

The CXR on ITU is taken AP, often with the patient supine or barely semi-erect, and is therefore difficult to interpret. On the ward the patient in bed leans back against the X-ray plate effectively holding it in position. The X-ray source is closer to the patient than for a departmental X-ray and therefore the incident X-rays are more divergent, causing magnification. In order to provide a normal erect orientation with the clavicles not overlying the apices, the incident X-rays are angled downwards. As a result, pleural fluid will not appear the same as it would on a truly erect CXR (*Figs 16.6* and *16.7*). See also *Section 4.4.1* on pleural disease and skin folds which may mimic pneumothoraces.

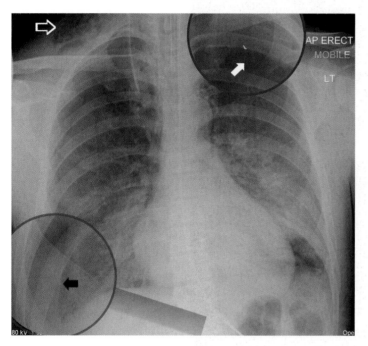

Figure 16.6. AP erect CXR.

Note the lung edge (white arrow) indicating the presence of a left pneumothorax. On the right in the magnified area there is another lung edge (black arrow) but with opacity beyond it indicating pleural fluid, but the density of this pleural effusion diminishes as you look further up. There is a hydro-pneumothorax on the right, but due to the semi-erect position of the patient, the air–fluid level is at an incorrect orientation to the incident X-rays to be seen. Note the further clue to the presence of a pneumothorax on the right is the surgical emphysema (open white arrow).

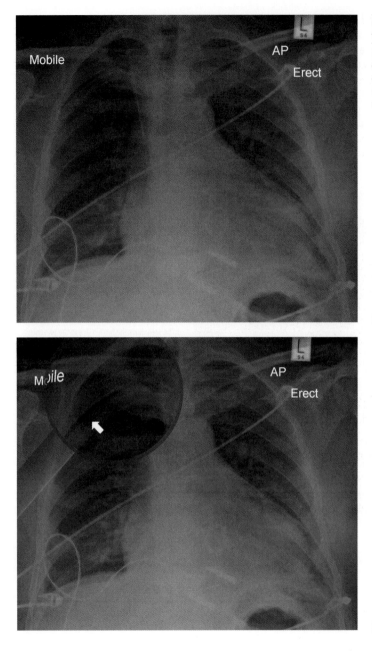

(a)

(b)

Figure 16.7. AP semi-erect CXR on an ITU patient following cardiac surgery.

(a) Note the epicardial pacing wires. The patient is off the ventilator but requiring greater amounts of oxygen than expected, can you see why?
(b) Same CXR with the right apical pneumothorax marked.

16.1 Adult respiratory distress syndrome

ARDS carries a poor prognosis and often requires a prolonged ITU stay during which the patient may be ventilated for long periods of time. The diagnosis is made clinically not radiologically. The appearances on CXR are of extensive bilateral consolidation extending to the peripheries, as opposed to the peri-hilar distribution seen in left heart failure. As these patients are invariably nursed supine or semi-erect, the consolidation is found in the dependent areas sparing the anterior aspect of the lungs. One of the problems in ARDS is the poor compliance of the lung, requiring high ventilation pressures which in turn may result in iatrogenic pneumothoraces (*Fig 16.8*).

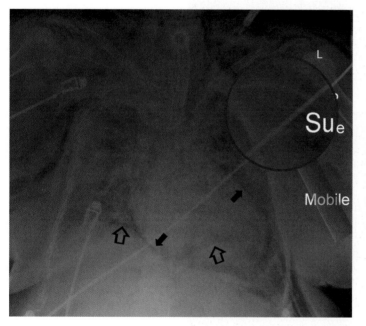

Figure 16.8. Supine CXR of an adult with ARDS being ventilated on ITU.

There is extensive consolidation, but this is dependent on site, sparing the anterior portion of the chest, hence the preservation of the hemi-diaphragmatic silhouettes (open black arrows). Note in the magnified area the streaky lucencies that correspond to free air within the pectoralis muscle. There is extensive surgical emphysema in the soft tissues of the chest and a pneumomediastinum (black arrows). There is clearly an air leak which could have originated from the tracheotomy site, but in this case there was a small pneumothorax; due to the poor lung compliance the lung was unable to collapse normally, allowing only a small pneumothorax but under a high pressure.

16.2 The CXR following thoracic surgery

Many ITU patients are being transiently cared for following surgery and are moved to less intensive care beds as soon as possible. Surgery involving the chest will inevitably have an impact on the appearance of the CXR (*Figs 16.9* and *16.10*). An awareness of the expected abnormalities on the CXR is vital if the unexpected abnormalities are to be recognised in what is, overall, a markedly abnormal appearing CXR.

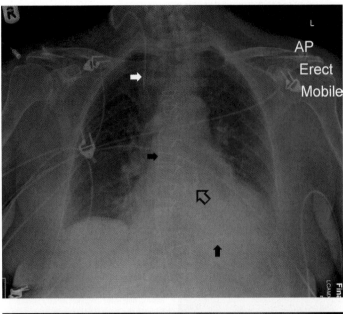

Figure 16.9. A typical AP CXR of an adult following cardiac surgery.

In this case the surgery was a tissue aortic valve replacement (open black arrow). Note the sternal wires, mediastinal drains (black arrows) and right internal jugular line (open white arrow). In addition, there is consolidation and collapse evident in the LLL and a small amount of pleural fluid is present. These are both routine findings in the post-sternotomy patient.

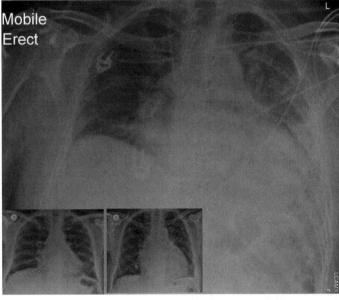

Figure 16.10. AP CXR day 1 after sternotomy, with inset CXRs before (left) and 9 days post-sternotomy (right).

Note the opacification at the left base due to a combination of pleural fluid and left lobe consolidation. These findings are not present on the pre-op. film and have resolved by day 9 post op.

Following sternotomy, the wires used to re-close the sternum should be visible. Note that there are non-radio-opaque closure devices available, but they are not in common use. These wires should be roughly in line as they are closing a straight wound; any misalignment of the sternal wires suggests wound dehiscence due to 'cheese-wiring' the sternal bone (*Fig. 16.11*). The wires may also fracture compromising the sternal closure (*Fig. 16.12*).

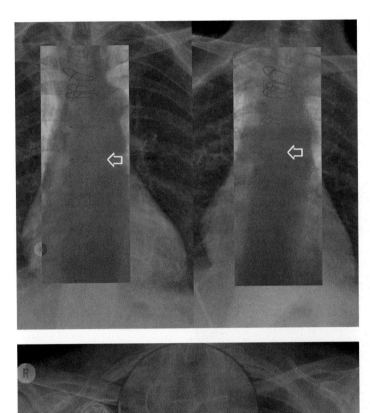

Figure 16.11. A portion of two AP CXRs of an adult following sternotomy.

Note the misalignment of the 5th sternal closure wire (open white arrow) on the right-hand image compared to the left-hand image; the sternal wound had dehisced.

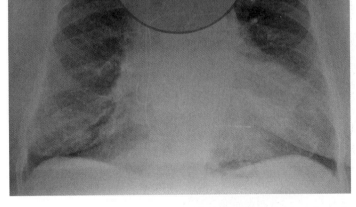
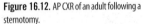

Figure 16.12. AP CXR of an adult following a sternotomy.

In the magnified area, the fragments of the manubrium sternotomy wire are seen due to the wire fracturing, leaving the sternal closure unstable.

The mediastinum following sternotomy will appear widened, partly due to the AP nature of the film, and therefore detecting significant mediastinal haemorrhage can be difficult; it often only becomes apparent when there is change in the post-operative mediastinal contour. In the early days following a sternotomy the LLL is usually collapsed and / or consolidated, but this should resolve with time and effective chest physiotherapy. A small to moderate pleural effusion is another common 'normal' finding following sternotomy and rarely requires intervention. As for the LLL pathology, the left pleural effusion should become progressively smaller – an enlarging pleural effusion or the presence of pleural fluid on the right should raise the possibility of fluid overload, left heart failure or possibly haemorrhage into the pleural space. Lung parenchymal abnormality other than in the LLL should be considered unexpected and is usually a result of impaired fluid balance. In the longer term, complications of sternotomy include a chronic left pleural effusion and paralysis / elevation of the left hemi-diaphragm due to phrenic nerve damage (*Figs 16.13* and *16.14*).

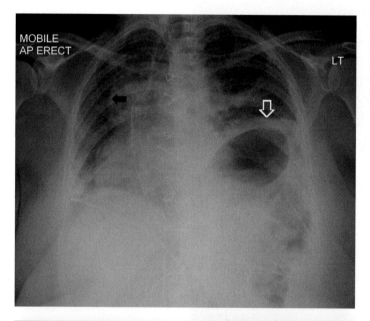

Figure 16.13. AP CXR 2 days following sternotomy for resection of a thymoma.

Note the elevation of the left hemi-diaphragm (open white arrow) due to damage to the left phrenic nerve during the procedure. There is also widening of the mediastinum (black arrow) suggesting mediastinal haemorrhage.

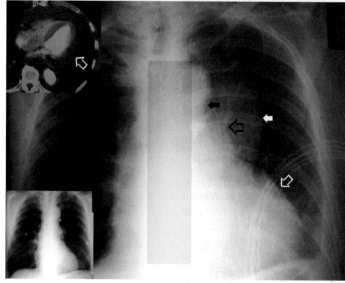

Figure 16.14. AP post-op. CXR and inset pre-op. CXR of an adult following a sternotomy.

Note the sternal wires in the contrast-enhanced area. There is a mediastinal mass (white arrow) not evident on the pre-op. film sparing the hilar silhouette (open black arrow), but obscuring the aorto–pulmonary window (black arrow). In addition, the cardiac contour has become more globular (open white arrow) when compared to the pre-op. film due to a haemopericardium following removal of the peri-operative epicardial pacing wires. This patient's complications were due to anticoagulant therapy.

17 The story films

The 'fun' way to approach the interpretation of a CXR is by treating it as the only clue in a solvable mystery. So, put on your deer-stalker, grip your elaborate pipe between your teeth and, wearing your very best Sherlock Holmes expression, have a look at the following CXRs. Each contains many clues to the underlying condition or sequence of events. The answers are at the end of the chapter. Good hunting.

Case 1.

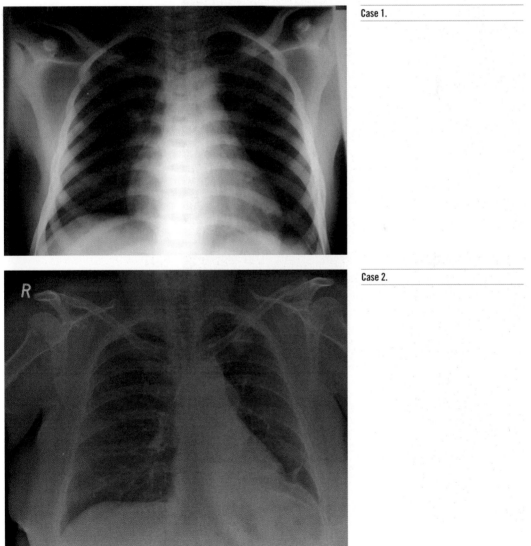

Case 2.

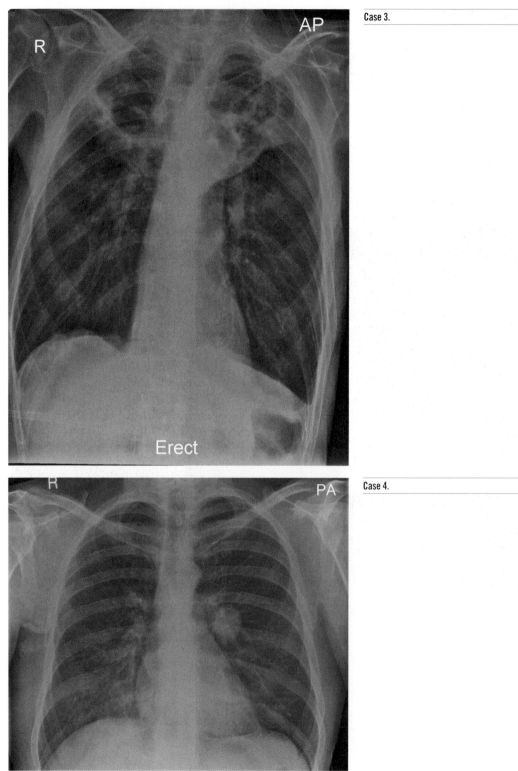

Answer to case 1

Sickle cell disease is a hereditary condition that results in a biochemical abnormality of haemoglobin; the abnormal haemoglobin crystallizes at low oxygen tension levels causing a change in the shape and flexibility of the red blood cells. Affected red blood cells cause embolisation of the small arterioles leading to end organ damage.

On CXR, the findings associated with sickle cell disease are cardiomegaly, atelectasis in the lung, sclerosis of the bones (see magnified area) and end plate depression of the vertebral bodies (see area of enhanced contrast).

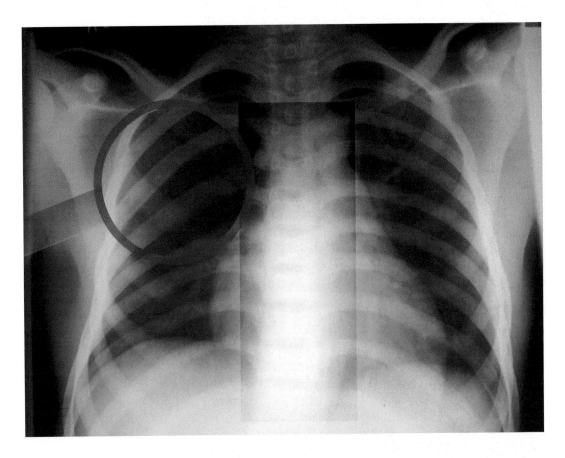

Answer to case 2

I hope you identified the nodule in the left apex (white arrow). In addition there is adenopathy in the aorto–pulmonary window (open white arrow). At this point this appears to be a peripheral tumour with A–P window adenopathy. However, loss of the medial left hemi-diaphragmatic silhouette (open black arrow) with increased density behind the heart and loss of volume at the left base (note the shift of the mediastinum), indicates LLL collapse. This last finding shifts the emphasis from a primary peripheral cancer to a central cancer causing LLL collapse with a metastasis in the left apex; synchronous primary cancers would be less likely.

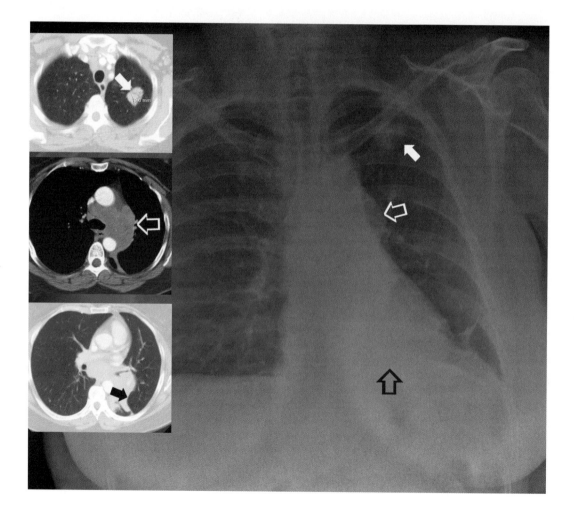

Answer to case 3

There are a few clues on this frontal CXR. In the smaller magnified area there is a radio-opaque coil, in the larger magnified area there is an IVC filter, and in both upper zones there is fibrocavitary disease most likely secondary to TB. The presence of the IVC filter indicates a history of pulmonary embolic disease where anticoagulation is contra-indicated; this helps explain the presence of the coil which, from its location, has been used to treat haemoptysis arising from the fibrocavitary disease in the right apex. The embolisation coil indicates a history of haemoptysis and, from its location, most likely originating from the fibrocavitary diseased lung.

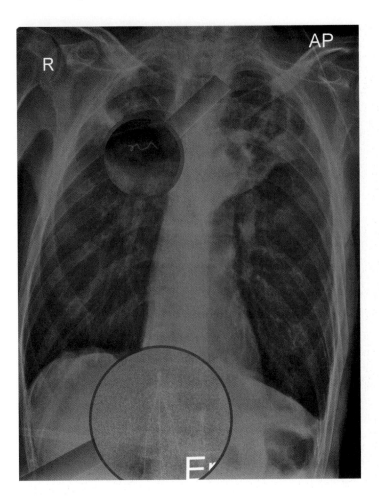

Answer to case 4

This patient has TB. The left hilar adenopathy (white arrow) and right lower zone consolidation (open white arrow) are relatively straightforward and should lean you towards infection rather than malignancy. The really tricky part is in identifying the air in enlarged lymph nodes at the right axilla (black arrow) and, even harder, the bony destruction of the scapula (open black arrow); compare the two sides. An infection from the lungs causing lymph node abscesses and osteomyelitis is most likely TB, although staphylococcal infection could also do this.

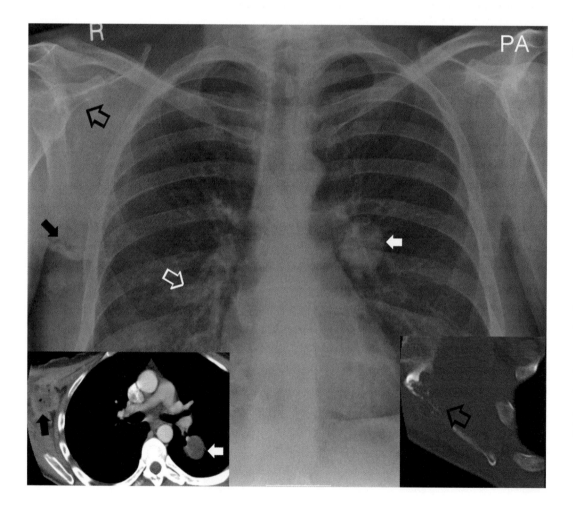

Further reading

Grainger RG, Allison DJ, Adam A, and Dixon AK (2008) *Diagnostic Radiology: a textbook of medical imaging, 5th Edition.* Churchill Livingstone, London.

Hansell DM, Armstrong P, Lynch DA, and McAdams HP (2010) *Imaging Diseases of the Chest, 5th Edition.* Mosby, New York.

Appendix

Answer to *Fig 3.2*

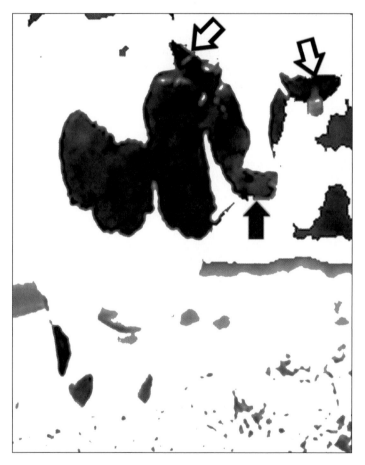

Figure. Answer to *Fig. 3.2.*

The image is that of a cow looking at you; the black arrow points to the end of its nose and the open arrows are pointing to the ears.

Answer to *Fig 3.7*

Expansive lesion in left seventh rib – an enchondrona.

Index

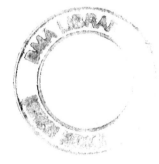